ANTI-FAT NUTRIENTS

Safe and Effective Strategies for
Increasing Metabolism, Controlling
Appetite, and Losing Fat in 15 Days

FOURTH EDITION

DALLAS CLOUATRE, PH.D.
with William Karneges

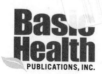

Basic
Health
PUBLICATIONS, INC.

The information contained in this book is based upon the research and personal and professional experiences of the authors. It is not intended as a substitute for consulting with your physician or other healthcare provider. Any attempt to diagnose and treat an illness should be done under the direction of a healthcare professional.

The publisher does not advocate the use of any particular healthcare protocol but believes the information in this book should be available to the public. The publisher and authors are not responsible for any adverse effects or consequences resulting from the use of the suggestions, preparations, or procedures discussed in this book. Should the reader have any questions concerning the appropriateness of any procedures or preparation mentioned, the authors and the publisher strongly suggest consulting a professional healthcare advisor.

Basic Health Publications, Inc.
8200 Boulevard East
North Bergen, NJ 07047
1-201-868-8336

Library of Congress Cataloging-in-Publication Data

Clouatre, Dallas, 1951–
    Anti-fat nutrients : safe and effective strategies for increasing metabolism, controlling appetite, and losing fat in 15 days / Dallas Clouatre with William Karneges.— 4th ed.
      p. cm.
    Includes bibliographical references and index.
    ISBN 1-59120-047-4
    1. Weight loss. 2. fat—Metabolism. 3. Vitamins. 4. Dietary supplements. I. Karneges, William. II. Title.

    RM222.2.C52 2004
    613.2'5—dc22

                                            2003028289

Editors: Stephany Evans and Tara Durkin
Typesetter/Book design: Gary A. Rosenberg
Cover design: Mike Stromberg

Printed in the United States of America

10   9   8   7   6   5   4   3   2   1

Contents

Acknowledgments

The authors would like to thank Dr. Jin-Bin Wu, Ph.D., of the College of Traditional Chinese Medicine in Taichung, Taiwan, for his generous contributions to this project. The authors would also like to thank Keiichi Morishita, President of the International Natural Medicine Society, for the donation of his work *The Theory of Food as the Main Factor of Cancer and Dietetics.*

Beyond Calorie Counting

This new edition of *Anti-Fat Nutrients* is similar in design and format to previous editions. As research progresses and new studies are done, however, we continue to increase our knowledge of how the human body works and how various nutrients work in the body. For this reason, important updates have been added to most sections.

"Dieting," that is, reducing caloric intake, was considered until recently to be the principal method for losing weight. At universities and nutritional research centers around the world this view is rapidly changing. A study by the National Institutes of Health suggests that there is no evidence that caloric restriction is a good *long-term* strategy for weight loss. In fact, for some people, cutting back on calories will lead to health risks.[1]

Certainly, those who significantly overeat can benefit from reducing their caloric intake. In general, however, calorie counting is not the solution to weight problems. Successful weight management requires a multifaceted approach involving nutrition, biochemistry, psychology, exercise, and lifestyle. Providing insight into some of these factors, this book will not only help you achieve greater weight control, but it also will help you look good and feel good.

Chapter 1 introduces new directions in the study of weight control and outlines the important contributions nutrients can make to dieters' lives.

Chapter 2 explores key nutritional supplements and the ways in which they facilitate weight loss.

Chapter 3 contains our Core Program, the Anti-Fat Nutrient Weight-Loss Program. This section also suggests specific nutrients that can help you not only control your appetite and lose weight but also reduce stress and relieve depression.

Chapter 4 covers the main elements of food and nutrition and offers dietary guidelines to help accelerate the weight-loss process.

Chapter 5 discusses the pitfalls of dieting as a method to control weight, reveals the real causes of obesity in America, introduces the importance of our metabolic individuality, and examines some of the most popular diets of the last century.

Chapter 6 sorts through the confusion surrounding the cholesterol issue and shows how nutrients can control cholesterol and help prevent heart disease.

Appendix: Nutritional Analysis of Foods is intended to be used in conjunction with Chapter 4. It also provides a handy reference to aid dieters in determining standard portion sizes and options for introducing into the diet more varied sources of protein, vegetables, and carbohydrates. Eating a broader range of foods is more healthful and tends to effortlessly reduce total caloric intake. This is especially true of vegetables, which are the best sources of "non-fattening" carbohydrates.

Although this book does discuss methods for reducing body fat and weight quickly, the primary aim of the authors is to help our readers make lasting changes in body composition and metabolism. To be a true success, a weight-loss program should provide the tools for achieving enduring good health. Therefore, dieters, resolve today to leave the "yo-yo" dieting pattern in the past! With the help of the following chapters, modify the foods you eat and the supplements you take to achieve permanent weight loss.

CHAPTER 1

Getting Lean through Nutrition

An estimated 97 million adults in the United States are overweight or obese, a condition that substantially raises their risk of morbidity from hypertension, dyslipidemia [the presence of elevated levels of total lipids in the circulating blood], type 2 diabetes, coronary heart disease, stroke, gallbladder disease, osteoarthritis, sleep apnea and respiratory problems, and endometrial, breast, prostate, and colon cancers. Higher body weights are also associated with increases in all-cause mortality. Obese individuals may also suffer from social stigmatization and discrimination. As the second leading cause of preventable death in the United States today, overweight and obesity pose a major public health challenge.

—EXECUTIVE SUMMARY OF CLINICAL GUIDELINES ON THE IDENTIFICATION, EVALUATION, AND TREATMENT OF OVERWEIGHT AND OBESITY IN ADULTS [NATIONAL HEART, LUNG, AND BLOOD INSTITUTE, 1999]

APPROXIMATELY 60 PERCENT OF ALL ADULT AMERICANS are over their ideal weight, and many more wish to slim down to look better and to lead more active lives. Unfortunately for most of the individuals who decide to diet, losing weight has become a yearly sparring match in which even an apparent knockout in the early rounds is followed by a reversal several months later. A large and thriving industry, one that sells several billion dollars a year in products and services, has grown up to take advantage of these difficulties, along with the desperation many face when they attempt to lose weight. This book provides do-it-yourself alternatives to empower dieters to achieve their ideal weight on their own. The following pages offer a compendium of current information on strategies for weight loss and on many of the products available to help those dieting take control of their lives and achieve the body weight they desire. In addition, some of the currently popular diets are explained and evaluated.

WHAT TO EXPECT

The end result of a successful weight-reduction program is more than merely the loss of excess weight. Many diets are initially effective for achieving rapid weight loss, but the weight is quickly regained once the diet is over because the pounds lost consisted primarily of water and lean muscle tissue. The result of the typical diet is that the percentage of the body's tissues made up of fats is increased and the percentage made up of the lean tissues that burn calories is decreased! The energy balances in the body are upset and future diets become more difficult because the body no longer responds. The typical diet, then, leads to a "yo-yo" pattern of weight loss–weight gain, with each cycle of weight gain usually more extreme than the previous one.

A successful diet does much more than simply take off unwanted pounds—it helps you feel good and look good. And it is permanent. This is because it includes making changes in body composition and metabolism that increase the body's ability to burn calories. These changes do not depend upon a large reduction in the calories consumed; rather, they rely on minor modifications in the foods eaten and on the addition of a small number of supplements to the diet. The result is a decrease in fatty tissue and an increase in the ratio of lean muscle tissue to adipose (fat) tissue in the body. Such a change is psychologically satisfying because lean tissue not only burns calories but also gives women their shapely figures and men their muscle tone. In any successful weight-loss program, you should be able to judge yourself by your mirror rather than by your bathroom scale!

THE VALUE OF WEIGHT-LOSS NUTRIENTS

Countless books have been written on dieting, exercise, and the psychology of overeating. Certainly these factors are important, but a significant area pertaining to weight control has remained relatively unexplored, namely, the nutritional biochemistry of weight loss. This book is unique because it offers an approach to weight loss that others do not: the means to a greater efficiency in fat metabolism. This is achieved through the proper use of what we refer to as "anti-fat nutrients."

Today millions of people worldwide are discovering the value that extra vitamins and other nutritional supplements can bring to their lives. For greater energy and healthier skin, as well as for prolonging life, vitamin and nutritional therapy is becoming recognized as the wave of the future. Now researchers are uncovering the roles that supplements can play in helping to control weight—from nutrients that increase the amount of fat that is burned for energy to nutrients that control sugar cravings. This book contains the latest scientific information on these anti-fat nutrients and offers a program to help you lose weight and improve your health in a safe and effective manner.

It has become apparent that "dieting" (restricting calories) is not a reliable solution to permanent weight loss. Although overeating may be the cause of weight gain in some individuals, many overweight people do not overeat. They are more likely the victims of inefficient fat metabolism and need an approach that addresses the efficiency of digestion, absorption, storage, and utilization of fat in the body.

Anti-fat nutrients are those nutritional substances that work at the biochemical level to reduce appetite and increase caloric expenditure. Some of these nutrients interfere with fat storage or increase the use of body fat as an energy source. Others, through a process called "partitioning," convince the body to use most of the calories consumed to feed lean tissues and for energy, rather than to add to fat stores. For thousands of individuals, the use of such anti-fat nutrients has resulted in weight loss and the increased ability to prevent new weight gain. After starting this program, dieters will experience greater energy and more control over their appetites. If you have a "sweet tooth," you will find that there are ways to undo cravings. Willpower is unnecessary when your biochemistry is brought into balance. Better yet, anti-fat nutrients encourage the burning of fat for sustained energy—unlike dieting, which encourages the loss of lean tissue.

The nutrients described in this book all have a variety of functions and benefits. L-carnitine, for instance, carries fat to the *mitochondria* in the cells. It is in the mitochondria that fat is burned for energy. However, the nutrient L-carnitine not only helps you get leaner, it also can help strengthen your heart and prolong life. This fact illustrates the power of nutrients: they tend to have many side benefits.

Certain nutrients are key factors in determining the body's tendency toward obesity or leanness. A truly effective weight-control program must address the issue of fat metabolism at the biochemical level. It must take into consideration not just calories but also the many factors that can impair fat metabolism. By choosing to include these nutrients in our diets, we can gain a measure of control over our individual metabolisms and have some say in whether our bodies gain or lose fat.

CHAPTER 2

The Anti-Fat
Nutrients

THIS CHAPTER CONSISTS OF IN-DEPTH DESCRIPTIONS of selected nutrients and metabolic categories. For each nutrient, we'll discuss its source and function, and give an overview of the research that has been done, along with any relevant data and results. We'll then explain how each should be taken for optimal results. In some cases, nutrients may have either cautions or side benefits, other than aiding weight loss; we will make you aware of these points as well.

The nutrients are listed alphabetically to enable you to find the discussion of the desired supplement quickly and easily. However, there is much value to be found even in the sections that may not match your immediate interests. Therefore, we encourage you to take a look at all the sections below and become familiar with the full array of fat-fighting substances. You may find that the actual research on a particular nutrient reveals that claims you have heard about it are overblown, and that it is really not of significant use for weight loss. On the other hand, you may discover one or more nutrients that were previously unknown to you, which may provide exactly the right support for your unique physical condition and diet.

ANTIOXIDANTS

Although most antioxidants are not specifically weight-loss agents (two exceptions being oolong and green tea), they may be important to dieters because they improve aspects of detoxification and energy metabolism. Strictly speaking, antioxidants are substances that remove from the body the byproducts of oxidative reactions and similar responses. A simple example of an oxidative reaction is our everyday metabolism. When the body burns food for energy, oxygen molecules from the air we breathe react with molecules of carbohydrates, proteins, and fats. If the chemical reaction is complete or "clean," then only water, carbon dioxide, and heat are produced. However, the burning process often is not complete—and even when it is, the oxygen that it requires will readily react chemically with parts of the body, not just food sources of energy. The result is the creation of what are known as "free radicals." A free-radical molecule is highly reactive because it has at least one unpaired electron that it seeks to balance by reacting with another molecule.

Free radicals damage the tissues in several ways. Perhaps the most direct is their attack on the membranes of cells. Cell membranes consist of proteins and lipids (fats). Free radicals can break the strands of proteins, cause the lipids to link to one another, and improperly bind the proteins and the lipids in other ways. This damage prevents cells from properly taking in nutrients and from properly removing waste products. The symptom commonly used to illustrate the results of free-radical attack on the membranes of cells is the loss of elasticity characteristic of aged skin. Yet damage to the wall of the cell is nevertheless preferable to mischief done within the cell itself, for free-radical activity inside the cell can alter the replication of the DNA and thereby initiate cancerous changes.[1] There are five basic types of damage caused by free radicals:

1. *Lipid peroxidation*—Free radicals initiate damage to fat-based compounds in the body. These compounds turn rancid and release yet more free radicals in a cascade.

2. *Cross-linking*—Free-radical reactions cause proteins and/or DNA molecules to fuse together. Protein-glucose cross-linking, a common type of damage found in diabetes, is particularly damaging.

3. *Membrane damage*—Free-radical reactions destroy the integrity of the cell membrane, which in turn interferes with the cell's ability to take in nutrients and expel wastes.

4. *Lysosomal damage*—Free-radical reactions rupture lysosome (cell digestive particle) membranes and allow the contents of the lysosomes to spill into the cell and digest critical cell compounds.

5. *Accumulation of the age pigment (lipofuscin)*—A buildup of lipofuscin (brown-pigmented, lipid-containing residues of lysosomal digestion) may interfere with cell chemistry.

Antioxidant nutrients are effective in neutralizing potential free-radical damage in two ways. First, they donate electrons to or combine with free radicals, thus preventing the free radicals from doing damage to the body's tissues. (The antioxidants themselves do not become chemically reactive after having scavenged free radicals.) Second, they are then either flushed from the body or restored back to their original condition.

Antioxidants come in three primary forms. The most important are enzymes that are produced by the cells themselves. These include superoxide dismutase (SOD), catalase, and glutathione peroxidase. Of secondary importance, but easier to use as supplements, are the nonenzymatic antioxidants, which are vitamins. These include vitamin A (and its precursor, beta-carotene), vitamin C, vitamin E, and a large number of less easily classifiable items, such as various flavonoids and polyphenols derived from citrus fruits, red wine, green tea, and so on. Also in this category are the substances L-carnitine and coenzyme Q_{10} (CoQ_{10}). A third category of antioxidants consists of certain minerals that are required in minute quantities; they include magnesium, manganese, selenium, and zinc. These minerals work mostly as cofactors of the vitamins and as actual components of the primary antioxidant enzymes.

For years, evidence has been accumulating which indicates that many antioxidants may improve the body's response to insulin. This has been demonstrated for the vitamins C and E, and for many of the flavonoids and polyphenols derived from fruits and vegetables. Tea catechins and similar compounds may also increase the rate of thermogenesis (see THERMOGENIC AIDS on page 73). Individuals who want to improve their blood sugar levels and their response to insulin might try taking 1–3 grams of vitamin C and a cocktail of other antioxidants, each day. For improving insulin response, however, the antioxidant alpha-lipoic acid is likely to be the best single supplement (see CHROMIUM, VANADYL SULFATE, AND OTHER INSULIN POTENTIATORS on page 23).

Controlling inflammation is another area in which some antioxidants excel. Excessive weight correlates to increases in the activity of reactive oxygen species (ROS) and dysregulation of immune functions, such as those of interleukin 6 (IL-6) and tumor necrosis factor-alpha (TNF-alpha). Human adipose tissue expresses and releases the proinflammatory cytokine IL-6, which leads to increases in C-reactive protein (CRP); hence, there are some clear pathways from obesity to chronically increased levels of inflammation. Some specialized plant extracts appear to be particularly successful in reducing such inflammation—probably more successful than the purified vitamin antioxidants. Green barley grass extract is one of the most powerful of such plant extracts. Several studies have demonstrated that the anti-inflammatory properties of this "natural SOD" are due to the ability of its micromolecular substances to scavenge ROS and to downregulate TNF-alpha production.[2]

All dieters should consider supplementing with alpha-lipoic acid. *The Merck Index* lists alpha-lipoic acid under the name *thioctic acid,* and it is under this name that most of the early research was conducted. The antioxidant role of alpha-lipoic acid was discovered only in 1988. For some thirty years previously, alpha-lipoic acid had been used primarily to treat the nerve damage that occurs in diabetes. It is now accepted that alpha-lipoic acid acts as a major antioxidant and as a scavenger of both water- and fat-soluble free radicals. This means that alpha-lipoic acid acts both inside cells and at the cell membranes. Alpha-lipoic acid scavenges hydroxyl radicals, singlet oxygen radicals, and, in the form of dihydro-lipoic acid, it scavenges peroxyl radicals as well as other radicals. It serves to either regenerate or spare both vitamin C and vitamin E. Some researchers consider it to be the "ideal antioxidant" or the "universal antioxidant."[3] It may be especially useful for maintaining metabolic functioning if supplemented in conjunction with acetyl-L-carnitine (see L-CARNITINE/ACETYL-L-CARNITINE on page 19).

How Antioxidants Help with Weight Loss

As a dieter loses weight, the body is forced to burn fats. To stay healthy while your body is burning fat at an accelerated rate, you should add antioxidants to your diet. Fat burning creates metabolic waste products. These include ketones (a breakdown product of fat oxidation) and lipid peroxides. Peroxides are dangerous free radicals. Perhaps even more damaging are the oil-soluble toxins and pesticides from the industrial environment, which collect in the body's fat stores. They include residues of DDT, PCBs, lindane, chlordane, and other noxious chemicals. These stored toxins are released as the dieter loses weight by burning fats. If exercise is a part of the diet process, they are removed from the body more easily. Many environmentally derived toxins are directly damaging to the body's ability to metabolize fats for energy, they promote the formation of free radicals, and so forth.[4] None of these waste products of fat metabolism (or toxins and pesticides released through the diet) will make the dieter feel better. On the contrary, they will interfere with weight loss and will certainly contribute to fatigue and other discomforts associated with dieting. By now there is a massive amount of research that indicates that supplements such as vitamins C and E are useful in controlling free radicals and preventing or treating ailments such as arthritis, cancer, diabetes, and heart disease.[5] The dieter should also be aware that the use of anorectics and thermogenic aids, both of which tend to speed up the body's metabolism, can increase the production of free radicals and therefore the need for antioxidants.

Very significantly, two powerful antioxidant extracts, those of oolong and green tea, by themselves can increase daily energy usage by 2.9 to 4 percent and increase the rate of fat oxidation by approximately 12 percent.[6] By themselves, these tea extracts will not lead to great weight loss in individuals who have difficulty controlling the amount of food they consume or who consume most of their calories late in the day. Nevertheless, oolong and green tea can help in diets of moderate caloric restriction and also aid in maintaining weight loss.

Availability and Usage

There are many nutrient formulas that include antioxidants among their vitamins and minerals. Those individuals undertaking rigorous and stressful programs such as dieting commonly find the addition to the diet of larger-than-RDA (Recommended Daily Allowance) amounts to be helpful. The RDA recently has been renamed and revamped once again to Percent Daily Value (%DV). Vitamin C usually is suggested at dosages of 1–2 grams a day in a nonacidic form divided among all the meals taken, whereas the %DV for vitamin C currently is 60 milligrams (mg) for most individuals. Vitamin E, which has a %DV of 30 IU (international units), is useful in dosages of approximately 200–400 IU, although as an oil-soluble vitamin it probably should not be taken in excess of 800 IU per day; like vitamin C, it should be cycled, that is, taken five days on and two days off, each week. Only the natural d-alpha-tocopherol and other more minor natural forms of vitamin E appear to be usefully active in the body as antioxidants.[7] (Synthetic vitamin E is usually listed as dl-alpha-tocopherol.) Indeed, research over the last decade has increasingly validated the role of gamma-tocopherol as the most active of the forms of vitamin E in protecting cell membranes and detoxifying what are termed "reactive nitrating species" of free radicals—types of free radicals that are particularly active in Alzheimer's disease and cardiovascular conditions. On the other hand, alpha-tocopherol often has been found to be ineffective.[8] Much recent research validates two points: First, natural vitamin E (d- rather than dl- forms) is more active than synthetic vitamin E. Second, of the four forms of vitamin E found in nature—that is, d-alpha-, d-beta-, d-delta-, and d-gamma-tocopherol—d-gamma-tocopherol has the widest range of benefits. Excessive ingestion of purified alpha-tocopherol, especially in its synthetic form, has the undesired effect of actually reducing the amount of gamma-tocopherol available to protect the membranes of the cells.

Dosages of the newer (and often far more powerful) antioxidants vary according to the manufacturers' instructions, your needs, and your budget. The extract of pine bark known as Pycnogenol, and the closely related grape seed extracts, are hundreds of times as powerful as vitamin C, but also many times more expensive. Furthermore, the absorption and effectiveness of some of the best antioxidants is greatly improved if these antioxidants are taken in conjunction with other substances. For instance, the highly potent bioflavonoid quercetin may be better absorbed by the body if taken on an empty stomach. Makers of barley grass extracts usually suggest that their products work best if taken between meals. Many in the health food industry argue that absorption of quercetin is improved by taking the proteolytic enzyme bromelain at the same time. (See DIGESTIVE AIDS on page 37.)

Antioxidants work best when they are used in conjunction with a well-balanced vitamin and mineral formula and with the proper diet. Some common and valuable antioxidants with suggested intakes are:

- Alpha-lipoic acid: 100–600 mg/day
- Beta-carotene: 1–25 mg/day; not suggested for those who consume alcohol
- Coenzyme Q_{10}: 10–150 mg/day
- Grape seed extract/pine bark extract: 100–300 mg/day
- Green tea extract: 500–2,000 mg/day
- Lutein: 3–30 mg/day
- Lycopene: 3–30 mg/day
- N-acetylcysteine: 100–750 mg/day
- Quercetin: 500–2,000 mg/day
- Selenium: 100–200 micrograms (mcg)/day

- Vitamin A: usually limited to no more than 10,000 IU daily
- Vitamin C: 150–3,000 mg/day
- Vitamin E (including especially gamma-tocopherol): 100–400 mg/day
- Zinc: 15 mg/day; zinc monomethionine is a preferred form

Note: The dieter who chooses to use large dosages of supplements of any sort and who later wants to cut back is advised to reduce the supplement(s) over a period of time to avoid any rebound effect. With most products, especially oil-soluble compounds, consider a cycle of five days supplementing, two days without supplements, each week.

APPETITE SUPPRESSANTS (ANORECTICS)

There are a number of natural appetite suppressants available both as supplements and through food sources. Foods that work to reduce hunger include fiber (see FIBER on page 46) and protein. Two supplements that act as anorectics, that is, as appetite suppressants, are the amino acids L-phenylalanine and L-tyrosine. (Note: Do not use the D- or DL- forms of these supplements for appetite suppression.) The thermogenic aids described later also can act as appetite suppressants. These include caffeine and the herb *ma huang,* a source of ephedrine (see THERMOGENIC AIDS on page 73). Similarly, natural lipogenesis inhibitors, which inhibit fat storage, generally double as anorectics (see LIPOGENESIS INHIBITORS on page 60). Just coming onto the market are pharmaceutical anorectics that work by preventing the storage of calories as fat.

It is sometimes suggested that the amino acid L-glutamine (not glutamic acid) can help to control sugar and alcohol cravings. The mechanism is unclear, although there is experimental support for the notion that an appetite control center in the brain is involved.[9] Glutamine in an animal test caused mice to lose 10 percent of their body weight, reduced blood sugar levels 50 percent, and reduced insulin levels 30 percent— even when the animals were fed a high-fat diet (45 percent fats). In a second experiment using a high-fat diet, the unsupplemented animals gained 15 percent in weight, yet the glutamine group gained no weight over a two-month period.[10] (See GROWTH HORMONE (GH) RELEASERS on page 54 for a more thorough discussion of L-glutamine.)

The anorectic herb wall germander (*Teucrium polium*) has been used in Europe, but it is not commonly available in the United States and there are questions now of liver toxicity if a related species of the herb is used.

Much more accessible are thermogenic herbs that also serve to reduce the appetite, such as green tea, kola nut, guarana, and ephedrine-containing plants.[11]

The hormone cholecystokinin (CCK) was available as an anorectic until 1985. CCK is an important key to appetite control. Since it plays a large part in the effectiveness of many of the other anorectics, it deserves some introduction. CCK is a hormone released from the hypothalamus, a section of the cerebral cortex of the brain. It is also released by the small intestine to stimulate digestion.[12] Significantly, it is one of the hormones that signal to us that we have eaten enough. Experiments have shown conclusively that injections of CCK into the proper area of the brain will prevent even starving rats from eating, whereas surgical damage to the hypothalamus to prevent the reception of the CCK stimulus will cause rats to eat themselves to death. Therefore, there is no doubt that this hormone is important in appetite control. However, appetite control induced by ingested CCK rapidly diminishes with chronic use.

A number of imitations of CCK are still being sold, but the real item is no longer available. CCK was considered a nutritional supplement until overzealous manufacturers made claims not yet validated according to U.S. Food and Drug Administration (FDA) regulations. These claims to druglike effects caused the FDA to pull all CCK from stores and prevent its future sale pending further clinical tests. Since CCK is a naturally occurring substance and therefore cannot be patented, it is highly unlikely that any company will ever put up the huge sums of money necessary to gain FDA approval. Since taking any hormone requires supervision, the setback with the FDA, in this particular instance, may not be such a terrible thing.

New appetite suppressants are appearing all the time. Some prove themselves to be effective and have staying power in the market, but most do not. One that works with food is the brand-name product Satietrol. This protease inhibitor, which is derived from potatoes, was shown to elevate CCK levels and to decrease food intake by 20 percent during an open-ended meal in normal-weight human subjects.[13] Habituation, at least over the short term, does not appear to be a factor with Satietrol. When taken in a beverage fifteen minutes before lunch and dinner, Satietrol led to weight loss of a little over 1 pound per week during a four-week trial.[14] Another product, Satise from Kemin Foods, appears to be a refinement of Satietrol. It actually quantifies the amount of potato-derived protein inhibitor (PI2).

Considerably less successful is an extract from jojoba meal called simmondsin. Based upon studies in rats and chickens, this substance appeared to be a nonstimulant regulator of the appetite, which, again, works by influencing CCK. Unfortunately, the large animal study was a disappointment,[15] and no tests have been performed in humans.

Recently, work has appeared on a mixture of herbs that successfully delays gastric emptying and thereby leads to weight loss. YGD is an herbal extract of yerbe maté (112 mg per capsule), guarana (59 mg), and damiana (36 mg). Three capsules are taken thirty minutes prior to lunch and dinner—or even breakfast, lunch, and dinner. Research has shown that with continued treatment, weight loss can be maintained for twelve months.[16]

In the future, it is likely that more "resistant" starches will appear as ingredients in meal replacements. These types of carbohydrates, which have been widely researched in Europe, release their glucose component much more slowly than do regular carbohydrates. Slow release means slow increase in blood sugar levels and more even release of energy.

Safe and effective supplements that can be used to stimulate the brain to release its own CCK, and which are available to consumers, are the related amino acids L-phenylalanine and L-tyrosine. L-phenylalanine is an essential amino acid. Through a series of biochemical reactions, L-phenylalanine is easily converted by the body to L-tyrosine. In turn, L-tyrosine is a precursor to a number of neurotransmitters and hormones, such as adrenaline (norepinephrine), dopamine, and thyroid hormones. This means that L-tyrosine is a precursor to important metabolism (including thermogenesis) stimulants and nervous system stimulants. L-tyrosine is a primary precursor to CCK in addition to having a weak antioxidant effect.

L-phenylalanine, the natural form of the amino acid, is recognized by the FDA as a food. (DL-phenylalanine, which is rarely found in nature, is a synthetic form.) As an amino acid, it is available through foods that have significant protein components, especially meats, poultry, and nuts. The presence of L-phenylalanine may be one of the routes by which high-protein diets serve to alleviate hunger in dieters. A number of special foods, such as spirulina, combine this essential amino acid with a variety of other benefits.

Spirulina has been used as a food by Central American and African tribes for centuries. It is now farmed and cultivated on a large scale in

California, Mexico, Japan, and elsewhere. It is sold around the world as a natural food supplement rich in nutrients. Over the last several years it has been discovered to be useful as an aid to weight loss. Spirulina contains substantial amounts of protein, essential fatty acids, vitamins, and minerals while also being low in calories. Experiments have shown that concentrated complete foods tend to reduce the appetite and partition energy into the body's lean tissues.[17] To date, nevertheless, there have been no clinical studies to specifically validate weight-loss claims made for spirulina. As a high-protein, low-calorie supplement taken between meals, spirulina undoubtedly will make sticking to a diet easier, but no special anorectic effects should be expected. However, aside from any weight-loss benefits, spirulina's virtues are many: it is a source of powerful antioxidants[18]; it may improve intestinal health[19]; and it can help to prevent the fatty liver[20] and abnormal levels of blood lipids induced by the consumption of excess fructose.[21] Fructose, the so-called fruit sugar (but now mostly extracted from corn), is often touted—wrongly and dangerously so—as being safe for diabetics.

Serotonin, which is produced from the amino acid L-tryptophan, is another neurotransmitter implicated in signaling satiety. The now-banned diet drugs fenfluramine and dexfenfluramine specifically targeted serotonin release and reuptake. This means that the drugs prevented the body from disposing of already "used" serotonin and thereby increased the amount of the neurotransmitter available to the nerves. Several still-legal supplements also increase available serotonin. Hence, a natural precursor to serotonin, such as 5-hydroxytryptophan (5-HTP), would appear to be a potential weight-loss aid.

Unfortunately, the amount of 5-HTP necessary to influence weight loss via appetite suppression seems to be quite high. Several Italian clinical trials have shown that 5-HTP in dosages of between roughly 600 and 900 mg per day, taken over periods of five to six weeks without dieting, can lead to weight loss averaging 3.1–3.7 pounds. (On diets restricted to 1,200 kilocalories per day, dieters lost between 6.8 and 7.3 pounds. The control group taking only placebo lost 1.1 pounds during the six-week trial.) Weight loss of half a pound per week without dieting is not a bad record. However, at the dosage level of 900 mg per day, 70 percent of the people in the 5-HTP group reported nausea during the first six weeks of the trials; the nausea did not continue into the second six weeks.[22] More recent trials with diabetic subjects also found benefit with 750 mg per day.[23]

Until these trials are repeated with much smaller doses, one must wonder whether the reported nausea induced at least part of the reported appetite suppression and weight loss. Likewise, at 750–900 mg per day, this product is quite expensive to use. Of course, 5-HTP may prove effective at much smaller dosages as an adjuvant to other diet aids. And at even smaller dosages, 5-HTP may prove helpful in controlling eating that is linked to stress and mood disorders. Furthermore, 5-HTP appears to be safe.[24]

Many individuals overeat for psychological reasons, such as depression or anxiety. Realistically, these dieters may benefit from herbs and nutrients to improve mood or otherwise reduce factors that trigger eating, especially binge eating. Moreover, those who are depressed or anxious often reduce, rather than maintain, their levels of physical activity. Hence, someone who eats to counter depression or who sits watching TV rather than taking a walk in the sunshine may find that treatment with S-adenosylmethionine (SAMe), the very significant mood elevator and liver protector, will ultimately have a greater impact upon his or her health and weight than a powerful appetite suppressant. *Rhodiola rosea* is an herb that has similar, but milder, effects upon mood and liver health.[25] A number of Chinese and Ayurvedic herbal formulas exist to improve mood and outlook (with herbs such as astragalus, ashwaganda, and others); these, too, might be given a try.

Other Benefits of L-Phenylalanine and L-Tyrosine[26]

- When taken over a period of time (that is, two weeks or more), both L-phenylalanine and L-tyrosine may help to control depression and anxiety.

- Both amino acids enhance learning, alertness, and memory.

- Phenylalanine in its "D" and "DL" forms is often effective for the control of chronic pain because these forms interfere with the degradation of endorphins (the body's own natural painkillers); however, these forms are less useful for appetite control.

- Phenylalanine/tyrosine use is sometimes associated with enhanced sex drive.

- L-tyrosine is a minor growth hormone (GH) stimulant.

- L-tyrosine is a precursor to thyroid hormones and may help correct mild hypothyroidism.

Availability and Usage

L-glutamine is available in many health food stores and should be taken on an empty stomach in dosages of 500 mg to 4 grams.

Since spirulina is a true food, it is quite safe and can be used like any other food. For dieting, however, best results come from taking this supplement either with breakfast or *instead of* breakfast, and then perhaps an hour before each of the other meals. Instructions come with the product, which can now be purchased in tablet form although it is usually found as a powder. At the start, a single dose might be half a teaspoon in a glass of water, and gradually increased to a full teaspoon taken two or three times a day. Also be aware that there are very large differences in quality between various brands of spirulina. The top grades can be quite expensive. Some cheaper grades of spirulina have undesirable bacterial counts, so it pays to find out about the quality of the product you are considering purchasing.

Both L-phenylalanine and L-tyrosine are available in 500-mg capsules, and the normal dosage is 1–2 capsules on an empty stomach. Many individuals can tolerate only smaller dosages at the start (see cautions below), so it is wise to begin with perhaps 250 mg or less and then increase the dosage. Since the body stores amounts of these amino acids, after a period of time it may be necessary to reverse this procedure and reduce the dosage. L-tyrosine is the faster acting of the two (the body produces L-tyrosine from L-phenylalanine after several hours), and it is commonly taken either before meals for better absorption or in the evening at bedtime a few hours after the last meal. Take these amino acids in the morning if your sleep is disturbed. L-tyrosine, but not L-phenylalanine, has been shown to markedly improve the appetite suppression found with ma huang (ephedrine).

Both L-phenylalanine and L-tyrosine require the presence of vitamins C and B_6 for conversion into several brain neurotransmitters. Therefore, it is important to supplement your diet with these vitamins for best results.

Cautions

Both L-phenylalanine and L-tyrosine can cause headaches, irritability, restlessness, and insomnia in sensitive individuals or at excessive dosages. Both can raise blood pressure, and they should not be used in conjunction with phenylpropanolamine (a common over-the-counter diet aid until the release of an FDA advisory in November 2002). They should never be used in conjunction with MAO inhibitor antidepressant drugs or in the presence of preexisting pigmented malignant melanomas (a specific skin cancer). If in doubt about the suitability of these products for your individual condition, always take the most conservative course and consult your physician or other licensed healthcare professional.

Since L-phenylalanine and especially L-tyrosine supply a substrate for the production of thyroid and adrenal hormones, they should be used with a bit of caution and in smaller quantities if taken in conjunction with thyroid and adrenal activators, such as ephedrine. Nevertheless, supplementation with L-tyrosine may help avoid the thyroid and adrenal exhaustion that is encouraged by the excessive and sustained consumption of caffeine and ephedrine, two items common in diet products that work primarily by increasing thermogenesis.

As indicated above, there is some concern regarding ephedrine, ephedrine/caffeine, ephedrine/caffeine/aspirin, and similar combinations, all of which are discussed later in this chapter (see THERMOGENIC AIDS on page 73). Also meriting concern are herbs with known or suspected toxicities, such as wall germander, which either itself, or certainly in variant species, is a liver toxin.

Artificial Appetite Suppressants

Natural anorectics usually are safe and effective for most individuals. These tend to work by supporting otherwise poorly functioning metabolic pathways, and this fact separates them from the drug appetite suppressants. Over-the-counter (OTC) appetite suppressants ("diet pills") contain various artificial chemical substances. Unlike the amino acid L-phenylalanine, which contributes to the production of the brain fuel norepinephrine (NE), the artificial phenylpropanolamine will, in about two weeks, deplete the brain reserve of NE. This reduction of NE produces a number of undesirable side effects including fatigue, depression, and other negative behavioral changes. Phenylpropanolamine recently was withdrawn from the market as an allowable OTC weight-loss preparation due to increased stroke risk; animal trials have shown evidence of liver toxicity. Other synthetic appetite suppressants include the drugs phentermine and fenfluramine; these drugs have serious side effects.

Dexfenfluramine, a more potent form of fenfluramine that is marketed as Redux, has recently become a focus of medical concern because studies suggest that it significantly increases the risk of pulmonary hypertension, a rare but often fatal lung disorder. Fenfluramine and its other derivatives (dexfenfluramine is classified as a derivative) also are implicated. Use for a period of three months or more increases the risk of pulmonary hypertension by thirty times.[27] There also have been reports that the use of dexfenfluramine in amounts only slightly above those commonly prescribed can lead to a radical reduction in the body's production of serotonin and even to the destruction of the cells that synthesize serotonin.

Sometimes items sold as "natural" weight-loss and appetite-control supplements, in fact, are laced with powerful drugs. Such items are often toxic to the liver. For instance, on July 21, 2002, there was a story widely reported on the Internet of Chinese slimming formulations, being sold into Japan, that caused liver and/or thyroid damage in a number of users. Some of these "herbal" products contained thyrotropic hormone; some actually contained dexfenfluramine. Similarly, in the United States in 2002 the "dietary supplement" LipoKinetix was withdrawn under FDA pressure after several instances of liver toxicity appeared. LipoKinetix, again, contained several essentially drug compounds that regulate thyroid function.[28] One can only caution here, "Let the buyer beware." Read labels and buy only reputable products from known sources.

A number of brain chemicals that suppress the appetite have recently been uncovered: leptin, glucagonlike peptide 1 (GLP-1), and the hormone urocortin. The primary site of action for most of these compounds is the hypothalamus. Thus far, these hormones and neurotransmitters have been shown to work only via injection. Drug versions of any of them are years away.

L-CARNITINE/ACETYL-L-CARNITINE

L-carnitine is an amino acid sometimes also known as "vitamin B-t." It is supplied in the diet primarily through animal muscle meats (from those of sheep and lamb, in particular), and it also is manufactured in the body, mainly in the liver and the kidneys. Produced from the essential amino acid lysine, the body's synthesis of L-carnitine requires vitamins C, B_6, and niacin, along with iron and the amino acid methionine. In humans, L-carnitine is concentrated in the heart and the skeletal muscles, and also in the brain and in the sperm.

Acetyl-L-carnitine (acetyl carnitine) is considered by many to be the most stable and bioavailable form of L-carnitine. It is involved in the same metabolic functions as is L-carnitine in its other forms, but acetyl-L-carnitine offers greater protections for the brain and neurons more generally. As an antioxidant, acetyl-L-carnitine protects neurons from damage caused by superoxide radicals. The molecular structure of acetyl-L-carnitine resembles that of the neurotransmitter acetylcholine. Recommended supplement amounts of acetyl-L-carnitine typically are about half that of other forms of L-carnitine. For most purposes, these compounds are similarly effective. However, research on preventing age-related mitochondrial decay and declines in mental abilities—perhaps even reversing some age-related mental declines—has stressed the combination of acetyl-L-carnitine and alpha-lipoic acid. This combination also appears to prevent the more generalized age-related decline in metabolic functioning.[29]

How L-Carnitine Can Help You Lose Fat

The primary role of L-carnitine in the body is as a biocatalyst. It serves to transport fatty acids across the membrane of the cell and into the mitochondria, where these fatty acids are burned for energy. It also aids in the removal of waste products from the mitochondria. (See "Hypothyroidism, Liver Function, and Brown Fat" on page 126 in Chapter 5.) L-carnitine, moreover, increases the rate of oxidation of fats in the liver, suggesting another way in which it improves energy generation.[30] Its impact upon fat metabolism is so sufficient that the *Physician's Desk Reference* has recommended dosages of 600–1,200 mg three times per day for the treatment of some forms of heart disease and some conditions involving elevated blood lipids.

There is no scientific doubt that a cellular deficiency of L-carnitine can lead to symptoms such as fatigue, muscle weakness, obesity, and elevated blood lipid and triglyceride levels. Moreover, carnitine itself is very safe, so supplementation may provide insurance in cases where there is question as to whether or not levels are sufficient. There are many anecdotal instances in which the supplement has helped to reduce excess weight. Jeffrey Bland, Director of the Bellevue Medical Laboratory, has argued that in the proper dosages, L-carnitine supplementation during dieting can help to control the negative effects of ketosis (the accumulation of waste products of fat metabolism) in those who are susceptible to this problem.[31] There is also evidence that some forms of obesity may be related to a genetic propensity to produce less L-carnitine; liver and kidney problems will similarly reduce the body's production, since some four-fifths of our L-carnitine total is produced internally by these organs.[32]

Finally, L-carnitine penetrates the mitochondria themselves. It is here that most free radicals are generated as food is oxidized to produce energy. There is some evidence that L-carnitine serves to spare antioxidants, such as vitamin C, although the mechanism by which this is done has not yet been uncovered.

Two caveats are in order. First, some researchers argue that increasing the level of L-carnitine in the system does not increase the rate or the amount of fatty acids used for energy except in cases where L-carnitine has been deficient, or in cases of special disorders. The experiences of healthy athletes with supplementation have been mixed. However, the results with healthy athletes are probably not appropriate for comparison with those of individuals suffering from excess weight or related difficulties. More important, current findings indicate that the mixed results came about because earlier researchers did not know what to look for and were not using the appropriate dosage levels.[33]

Second, a few authorities recommend that L-carnitine not be taken in instances of active kidney or liver disease. This caution is a matter of dispute inasmuch as other authorities actually suggest that supplemental L-carnitine aids in the treatment of some forms of kidney malfunction. However, those with active liver or kidney disease and those with diabetes or a propensity toward diabetes should follow a conservative course of action and consult a physician.

The big question for dieters, of course, remains: Does supplementing with L-carnitine lead to greater weight loss? The answer is, taken by itself without any changes in diet, probably not much. Animal studies have shown, however, that in conjunction with a mild reduction in caloric intake, L-carnitine can quite significantly improve the weight lost on a diet program over a period of many weeks.[34] Therefore, use this supplement in conjunction with some form of mild caloric restriction, and do not expect to lose pounds merely by taking L-carnitine alone.

Other Benefits of L-Carnitine

- Reduces fatigue.

- Can be used therapeutically in the treatment of atherosclerotic heart disease.

- Increases the levels of HDL (the desirable high-density lipoprotein cholesterol) in the blood while decreasing the levels of triglycerides and LDL (low-density lipoprotein) cholesterol.

- Reduces ketone levels in the blood.

- May increase the motility and the fertility of sperm.

- May improve liver performance in cases of alcohol abuse.

- May improve some forms of kidney disease.

Availability and Usage

L-carnitine is available in 250-mg capsules at most health food stores. Some companies supply 500-mg capsules as well. The dosage should always be taken on an empty stomach. Liquid L-carnitine is also available, but some people find the glycerin base to be too sweet. Liquids tend to speed up absorption, but are not necessarily as stable or as tolerable as capsules and tablets. The dosages commonly suggested for improved fat metabolism are 1,000–5,000 mg daily in separate doses. To prevent the possibility of developing a tolerance at these dosage levels, it is advisable to discontinue taking L-carnitine for several days each month. *Only the L- form of carnitine should be taken, never the D- or DL- forms, which have side effects.*

People whose livers and kidneys are functioning properly can effectively increase their L-carnitine levels by increasing their consumption of lysine-containing foods (especially fish and the dark meat of poultry) and by adding to their diets vitamin C and the other nutrients needed for carnitine production. One study showed that adding as little as 200 mg of vitamin C to the daily diet increased L-carnitine synthesis in the body. If supplemental lysine is taken, 500 mg–1 gram total in divided doses taken daily before meals has been recommended. Supplementation with vitamin B_5 (pantothenic acid or preferably its active coenzyme form, pantethine) improves the action of carnitine by increasing the production of acetyl-CoA in the body. Research suggests that carnitine works synergistically with coenzyme Q_{10} and pantethine. Also, supplementing with choline (20 mg per kilogram of body weight) may reduce urinary L-carnitine losses by as much as 75 percent.[35]

CHROMIUM, VANADYL SULFATE, AND OTHER INSULIN POTENTIATORS

As you will see in Chapter 5, problems in carbohydrate metabolism play a large causative role in the American tendency to put on excess weight. One of the primary substances involved in fat storage is the hormone insulin, so it is reasonable to presume that foods and nutrients that make insulin more effective and that mimic insulin's actions in the body might aid in controlling appetite and weight gain. An enormous amount of scientific attention is now being directed toward a number of micronutrients that appear to perform just these functions. Among these are the trace minerals chromium and vanadium, the Ayurvedic herb *Gymnema sylvestre,* and some cooking herbs and spices, including bay leaves, "apple pie spice" (allspice), cinnamon, cloves, and turmeric. The mechanisms by which these work vary.[36] We will discuss each of these different insulin potentiators individually.

CHROMIUM

Of the insulin potentiators, chromium has been the subject of the most study because, in 1957, it was discovered to be central to a substance known as glucose tolerance factor (GTF). GTF is made up of one form of chromium—the mineral in its trivalent state—combined with niacin and the amino acids glycine, cysteine, and glutamic acid. Unfortunately, no one has yet learned how to manufacture or extract GTF, and chromium itself is difficult for the body to manipulate into its biologically active form.[37]

Chromium, as part of GTF, is thought to improve the absorption of glucose into the cells, making it more useful for energy. Since GTF also potentiates the effects of insulin (makes insulin more effective), less insulin is needed and blood sugar levels are stabilized. This means that energy levels also are stabilized and the extreme fluctuations of hunger associated with hypoglycemia are avoided. The usefulness to the dieter and to those with diabetic tendencies is obvious. Just as important, however, is the fact that chromium has been shown to help decrease unwanted blood lipid levels, both of low-density lipoprotein (LDL) cholesterol and of triglycerides, while actually raising the levels of high-density lipoprotein (HDL), the desirable cholesterol, in the blood.[38] Many of the actions given below for vanadium also apply to chromium and other insulin potentiators; so, with important exceptions, these substances are interchangeable.

The American diet is notoriously deficient in chromium, and it is commonly estimated that as many as 90 percent of all Americans are marginally deficient in chromium or worse. We certainly suffer in comparison with parts of the world in which diabetes and heart disease remain rare. In most parts of Asia, tissue levels of chromium are five times higher than in the United States.[39] Similar low tissue levels are true of Americans tested for many other important minerals, and two likely causes are our farming methods and our processing and refining of many foods.

The evidence that chromium supplements can lead to weight loss is quite contradictory and controversial. It is quite well established that insulin resistance (Syndrome X, also called the metabolic syndrome) is strongly causally linked to the development of obesity and that the correction of insulin resistance is therefore necessary for long-term dieting success. However, this does not mean that improving insulin response by itself will in the short term lead to weight loss. Clinical experience bears out this point. Improving insulin response is always a good idea with regard to health, but no one should expect the pounds to melt away merely because he or she is supplementing with chromium.

VANADIUM

Current interest in the trace mineral vanadium dates to 1985, when an article in the prestigious journal *Science* indicated that vanadium controlled diabetes in laboratory animals.[40] This data created excitement because it showed that vanadium is effective when taken orally—in contrast to insulin, which must be injected to be effective. Other studies quickly confirmed these results, and it is now known that vanadium plays an important role not only in controlling blood sugar levels, but also, as is true of chromium, in preventing the development of excessive levels of LDL cholesterol and triglycerides.[41] Further evidence exists to the effect that vanadium assists in the development of the bones and teeth.

These impressive findings actually constituted a rediscovery of the uses of vanadium. In France, vanadium was already a medically recommended treatment for diabetes and some forms of fatigue in the late nineteenth century. In the English-speaking world, the 1932 edition of *Dorland's Medical Dictionary* listed vanadium as a treatment for diabetes and neurasthenia; with the addition of selenium, it was also suggested as a treatment for cancer. In the 1958 edition of *Dorland's*, atherosclerosis (hardening of the arteries) was added to the illnesses for which vanadium was recommended. Vanadium therefore has a track record of usage by human beings, not just of tests on laboratory animals.

Although not as successful as injected insulin for the treatment of extreme cases of diabetes (which is the reason that it originally disappeared from medical usage), vanadium in the form of vanadyl sulfate (its biologically active form) can mimic many of the activities of insulin. In this respect, vanadyl sulfate is even more impressive than chromium. Chromium potentiates the body's insulin, but the vanadyl form of vanadium itself is biologically active even in the absence of insulin. It significantly increases liver glycogen (stored glucose) and it improves the uptake of glucose by muscle tissues. These actions help to spare lean tissue during dieting and to improve athletic performance by lessening fatigue and reducing the breakdown of muscle protein for energy. Vanadyl sulfate thus possesses "anti-catabolic" properties, that is, it acts to prevent tissue breakdown. Nevertheless, it also acts to inhibit the storage of excess calories from carbohydrates as fat, apparently by stabilizing the body's production of insulin. These properties, again, are useful for controlling weight gain and for improving athletic performance.

All of this sounds very good, but there are at least two major caveats regarding vanadium compounds. First, especially in the presence of aluminum, vanadium is a promoter of free-radical generation.[42] The pro-oxidant properties of vanadium compounds are well known. Second, and likely as a result of vanadium's pro-oxidant properties, especially in fats, very high intakes of vanadium compounds have been associated with elevated liver enzymes. Such reports typically have involved intakes of 50–60 mg of vanadyl sulfate per day. Recent studies suggest that side effects (gastrointestinal, liver, and kidney) are not found with organic vanadium compounds, and therefore the future of vanadium supplements clearly lies with these newer and safer forms.[43]

GYMNEMA SYLVESTRE

The herb *Gymnema sylvestre* has been used in Ayurvedic medicine for two millennia to control problems in carbohydrate metabolism. Animal studies have confirmed that the herb does indeed reduce blood sugar levels.[44] Other studies demonstrate that *Gymnema sylvestre* extracts increase the functions of the liver and the pancreas, areas which tend to have weakened functions in those who are overweight. Another factor of significance to dieters is the fact that *Gymnema sylvestre* appears to reduce cravings for sweet foods,[45] and it does this by affecting the taste receptors.[46] As with chromium and vanadium, this insulin potentiator appears to normalize blood lipid levels and to lower insulin requirements. However, unlike the two micronutrients, *Gymnema sylvestre* may work by repairing and/or regenerating the insulin-producing cells of the pancreas, thereby increasing the output of insulin.[47]

A late addition to the list of blood-sugar-regulating supplements is a product commonly sold under the brand name Glucosol. Derived from the herb *Lagerstroemia speciosa* L., otherwise known as crepe myrtle, the banaba tree, or colosolic acid (the active agent in Glucosol) is a relatively newly discovered glucose-disposal agent. Colosolic acid has been shown to lower blood levels of glucose in humans.[48] This effect previously had been shown in hyperglycemic animals.[49] From in vitro studies, colosolic acid appears to work by stimulating the cell's glucose transporters.[50] Another interesting finding is that colosolic acid may be useful in weight loss.[51] This is not true of many compounds that help to regulate blood sugar levels. For instance, although trivalent chromium may be useful as part of a weight-loss program, its weight-loss benefits, if chromium is taken alone, are quite weak. Anecdotal feedback would support significant weight-loss benefits in roughly one-third of those using colosolic acid for this purpose.

Benefits of Insulin Potentiators

- Control blood sugar levels and thereby affect energy levels and hunger spikes.

- Help to normalize fat storage and improve utilization of fat for energy.

- May help to increase lean tissue in the body and to "build muscles" in those who actively train with weights.

- May help to prevent and to control diabetes.

- Chromium and vanadium lower blood lipid levels, and chromium may raise the level of HDL, which is desirable.

- Chromium and vanadium may strengthen the immune system.

- Vanadium plays a role in the laying down of calcium in the bones and teeth.

Availability and Usage

Chromium is not well absorbed by the body, and there is presently enormous controversy as to which form of chromium supplement is best assimilated. Most of the research showing significant effects has been done with the picolinate or polynicotinate (ChromeMate) forms, and the consensus seems to be that, of the least expensive forms available, these may be the best. Both chromium picolinate and polynicotinate are sold by most of the leading vitamin companies. Since absorption is poor for almost any form, 200 mcg is likely a safe long-term dosage for any individual. Therapeutic dosages may be as much as 1,000 mcg per day, although such a high intake probably should not continue for more than a few months without a break. *Only the trivalent form of chromium should be taken.*

Currently there is no accepted Recommended Daily Allowance (RDA) for vanadium, although it is recognized that a deficiency of this trace mineral is detrimental to both animal and human health. The average diet provides roughly 2 mg of the elemental form per day from fats and vegetable oils, and in some parts of the world (particularly in areas of South America) diets provide 10–15 mg of elemental vanadium per day, which is quite high. Absorption is usually only about 5 to 10 percent of that ingested, and the unused amount is readily excreted. The recommended supplemental dosage of vanadyl sulfate is 1–2 mg per day, and more for special purposes. Some studies have used 22.5 mg of vanadyl sulfate per day for sixteen months without toxic effects, but others report that this amount is actually in excess of what can be absorbed, and that no further benefits can be expected in dosages over 15 mg per day (with the exception of diabetics under medical supervision). In other words, there is no consensus on effective dosage levels. The vanadate forms of vanadium should not be taken as supplements.[52] A new form of vanadium, bis(maltolato)oxovanadium(IV), has recently been developed that is both more potent and even safer than vanadyl sulfate, and other specifically organic forms of vanadium are being researched. (See also the previous remarks under "Vanadium" regarding the pro-oxidant properties of vanadium compounds at excessive intakes.)

Gymnema sylvestre is sometimes included in diet formulas for its effect upon the perception of sweetness. However, this is of somewhat questionable benefit to most individuals. The more appropriate use of the herb is for its insulin-potentiating effects and its effects upon the liver and pancreas. For these purposes, the whole herb should probably be used. The

Indian common name for the plant is *shardunika*. Dosage depends upon the extract, but can run to several hundred milligrams per day.

Glucosol (crepe myrtle extract) usually is supplemented at the rate of 48 mg per day—a rather compact dosage form.

Some of the most potent regulators of insulin also are the most pleasant to use. Good-quality cinnamon, although not inexpensive, is very useful in this regard, as are allspice, cloves, and turmeric (curcumin). Turmeric has the added advantage of being a liver detoxifier and an anti-inflammatory. Bay leaves, although too strong to use in great quantity, improve digestion of legumes and fats and have been used since ancient times for their healthful properties.

Cautions

There is a clinically recognized form of depression that is treated with a low-vanadium diet. This syndrome is genetic and not vanadium induced, but someone being treated for depression should consult his or her physician before adding vanadium to the diet. Those taking MAO inhibitors should not take vanadium supplements. Corrections of elevated blood glucose levels also may leave one *temporarily* tired. This may result from the use of insulin potentiators and mimics.

Some insulin-resistant individuals may find that *Gymnema sylvestre* increases insulin levels too much, which can elevate blood pressure in rare cases. These individuals should employ other insulin potentiators to improve their insulin sensitivity.

COENZYME Q_{10} (CoQ$_{10}$)

Coenzyme Q_{10} (CoQ$_{10}$), also called "ubiquinone" because it is present in nearly all cells, is obtained from the diet (mainly from fatty fish, organ meats, and whole grains) and is also produced by the body. Some have suggested that CoQ$_{10}$ will soon be classified as an oil-soluble vitamin because it is now known to be essential and because its deficiency leads to health problems. Chemically, its structure is related to that of the vitamins E and K. The amino acid methionine is essential for its production. CoQ$_{10}$ appears to be virtually nontoxic.

CoQ$_{10}$ is similar to L-carnitine in that it is important chiefly for its role in the mitochondria, the intracellular organelles that produce energy. The important energy-storage chemical ATP (adenosine triphosphate) is produced by the mitochondria with the aid of CoQ$_{10}$. The coenzyme is also a potent antioxidant, as its structural similarity to vitamin E suggests. It scavenges free radicals by donating its own electrons, and it also helps to prevent lipid (fat) peroxidation.[53]

How CoQ$_{10}$ Helps with Weight Loss

As with L-carnitine, CoQ$_{10}$ may prove beneficial to those who are overweight because it improves the efficiency of energy production at the cellular level. There is some evidence that certain inefficiencies are related to genetic inheritances concerning the body's ability or inability to manufacture this coenzyme. About half of those with family histories of obesity do not respond to the ingestion of food as they should. A normal response to a meal is for the body to slightly raise its rate of energy production. Many of those who are overweight do not have this response. Blood serum tests for levels of CoQ$_{10}$ indicate deficiencies in almost 50 percent of the obese subjects.[54]

Clinical trials specifically designed to evaluate CoQ$_{10}$ as a weight-loss agent are lacking. However, there is some evidence that this quasi-vitamin can improve pancreatic beta-cell response and glycemic control in pre-diabetic and diabetic individuals.[55]

Other Benefits of CoQ$_{10}$

- Under the proper conditions CoQ$_{10}$ significantly improves athletic endurance.[56]
- CoQ$_{10}$ is used in Japan and elsewhere to treat congestive heart failure, cardiac arrhythmias, and ischemic injury.[57]
- CoQ$_{10}$ is effective for lowering blood pressure.
- The coenzyme has been found to serve as an immune stimulant that boosts the capacities of existing immune cells. It may reduce the toxic side effects of chemotherapy.
- Periodontal disease has been improved or even reversed with daily dosages of 50–70 mg.

Availability and Usage

CoQ$_{10}$ is a relatively expensive supplement, or at least it has been until quite recently. It is commonly available in 10-mg, 30-mg, and 60-mg capsules. The effective amount is usually 10–20 mg, taken two or three times a day, although therapeutic dosages with heart patients have been as high as 150 mg per day for four weeks or longer. Amounts of up to 100 mg a day have been taken by Japanese consumers for extended periods of time with only positive effects, so the safety of the coenzyme is well established. In Japan over 15 million people, about 10 percent of the entire population, take this coenzyme regularly. Some researchers suggest that additional benefits accrue if CoQ_{10} is supplemented with vitamin E daily along with other basic nutrients. Experimental results demonstrate that oral supplementation with alpha-tocopherol (vitamin E) alone results in serum LDL (low-density lipoprotein) that is more prone to oxidation initiation, whereas co-supplementation with coenzyme Q_{10} not only prevents this pro-oxidant activity of vitamin E, but also provides the lipoprotein with increased resistance to oxidation.[58]

CONJUGATED LINOLEIC ACID (CLA)

Conjugated linoleic acid (CLA) is a fatty-acid nutrient that occurs naturally in beef, turkey, and many dairy products—but only if the animals had adequate access to grass or green silage rather than having been raised primarily on grain. This nutrient was discovered in the mid-1980s by researchers who found that beef exerted an unexpected anticancer effect. Further investigations indicated CLA's function as an immune-system modulator, which means that it alters some immune functions and how the body reacts to immune stimulation. As a rule, overactivation of the immune system can lead to the loss of lean tissue, yet animals fed CLA in trials did not suffer from wasting or other adverse effects to the same extent as those in control groups when they were injected with toxins or certain types of vaccines.[59]

Currently, scientists believe that CLA alters the way in which fats are metabolized and stored in various membranes and tissues. The ratio of saturated fats to monosaturated fats in tissues is increased with the ingestion of CLA. The result of this change in several species of animals studied is a reduction in food consumption, a reduction in stored fat, a better ratio of high-density lipoprotein cholesterol (HDL, the "good" cholesterol) to low-density lipoprotein cholesterol (LDL), a better ratio with regard to total cholesterol, and a reduction in atherosclerosis.[60]

Originally, CLA was available only from animal sources. However, now CLA can be produced commercially from sunflower seed oil.

How Does CLA Work?

CLA has shown its best results when examined as a protective agent against cancers and as a modulator of immune function. Under challenging conditions, CLA prevents the catabolism (tissue breakdown) that accompanies excessive immune stimulation.[61] CLA also apparently changes, to some extent, the metabolism of lipoproteins (fats carried in the blood via protein packets) and the manner in which the body utilizes fats for energy. In animal studies, CLA reduced overall food consumption as well as the percentage of weight as fat, hence the animals were leaner. Another way of describing the actions of CLA is to call it a partitioning agent,[62] which is to say that it changes the balance of lean to fat tissue and the ratio of ingested energy that the body allocates to different types of tissues. In part this reflects, at least in one animal model, greater energy expenditure.[63]

There is some experimental evidence that CLA helps to prevent the development of insulin resistance,[64] as well as increases in body fat.[65] A much greater body of evidence from animal studies indicates that this supplement can improve lean-to-fat ratios in the body.[66] It should be pointed out that the results of trials have varied dramatically from species to species. Many of the studies done to date have focused on CLA's benefits for improving lean weight gain in animals eating less food.[67] What reports we have show a similar pattern of benefits for humans. The subjects became leaner, but not lighter. This may be important to dieters, in that long-term stress and just plain aging are known to lead to weight gain through a reduction in lean body mass. Hence CLA may be important for maintaining leanness, including in aging individuals, but not significant by itself for helping the overweight to lose pounds. The authors are unaware of any published clinical trials proving weight loss utilizing CLA.

Another Benefit of CLA

Another potentially health-enhancing benefit of the consumption of supplemental CLA, especially in conjunction with the omega-3 fatty acids EPA (eicosapentaenoic acid) and DHA (docosahexaenoic acid), is an inhibition of the cyclooxygenase-2 (COX-2) enzyme.[68] This enzyme is important to the synthesis of arachidonic acid. As a result, it plays an outsized role in the generation of reactive oxygen species (ROS) and the promotion of inflammation. By inhibiting cyclooxygenase, CLA in conjunction with EPA and DHA helps to reduce the activity of processes that increase inflammation.

Availability and Usage

Only recently has CLA become available at prices appropriate for a nutritional supplement. CLA is an oil and is supplied primarily in capsule form. Its makers usually recommend taking 3,000–6,000 mg of CLA per day in divided doses. Most dieters should use the higher dosage.

DEHYDROEPIANDROSTERONE (DHEA)/7-KETO-DHEA

Dehydroepiandrosterone (DHEA) is the primary steroid hormone produced by the adrenals and, in small amounts, by the testes. It possesses about 5 percent of the androgenic effect of testosterone. The body's production of DHEA increases until sometime in a person's twenties to a level of between 7 mg and 15 mg of new production per day, and then declines gradually. By the age of sixty, blood levels of the hormone typically are only two-thirds of early adulthood levels. By the age of eighty, DHEA blood levels may have declined by 95 percent. Most of the DHEA within the body is found in the form of DHEA-S, that is, DHEA that has had a sulfate molecule attached to it by the liver. It is generally considered to be less active than DHEA in most physiological processes. It may be possible to increase DHEA blood levels through dietary manipulation, but DHEA supplementation is best achieved with pharmaceutical-grade materials.

Technically, DHEA is a "pro-hormone" rather than an active hormone. It is the precursor to the steroid hormones of the body, including estrogen, progesterone, cortisone, testosterone, and other steroid and sex hormones. DHEA can be converted to these otherwise difficult-to-construct hormones as needed, and any excess is typically excreted.[69]

3-acetyl-7-oxo-dehydroepiandrosterone, also known as 7-keto-DHEA, is one of several metabolites of DHEA. It is said to be safer because, unlike DHEA, it does not serve as a hormone substrate. At least in the short term, this appears to be true.[70]

How Does DHEA Work?

Besides providing the building blocks for many of the body's most important hormones, DHEA works by inhibiting an enzyme called G-6-PD (glucose-6-phosphate dehydrogenase), which serves to store fat. The unstored fat is then either shunted into energy pathways or excreted. It has been recognized that obese individuals excrete less DHEA through the urine than do non-obese individuals; this suggests that obese individuals are producing much less of this pro-hormone. Douglas L. Coleman and

Edward H. Leiter of the Jackson Laboratory of Bar Harbor, Maine, have found that very large doses of DHEA can apparently block or even reverse the effects of the genes responsible for obesity and diabetes in experimental animals. The blockage of G-6-PD may also explain the anti-tumor activity of DHEA in both animals and humans.[71]

DHEA is known to increase the insulin sensitivity of cells, an important factor in both diabetes and obesity. It also increases sensitivity to thyroid hormone, thus improving thermogenesis, fat metabolism, and energy production. Finally, it improves liver function, thus ameliorating a weakness common to obese individuals.[72]

Unfortunately, animal models and experiments have yielded results that too often have not been reproduced in human trials. The clearest case is that of obesity, although there is quite a bit of controversy on this point. DHEA works extremely well in controlling obesity in rodents. Most human obesity trials, however, have proven successful only at very high levels of intake (1,500 mg per day). Nevertheless, there is no doubt that DHEA is active against a range of conditions. Several medical articles published in 1997, and which were based on small trials, seemed to indicate that elderly patients who are given DHEA respond more favorably to flu vaccine. However, subsequent elaborate trials have not supported this claim.[73] Claims of benefits to elderly subjects from supplementation with DHEA in terms of mood, quality of sleep, and so on, although initially promising, also have received little support from vigorous testing, albeit cognitive improvements continue to be reported. DHEA supplementation, therefore, remains controversial.[74]

The human clinical evidence of DHEA's antiobesity potential is spotty, although there is some data that suggests the hormone has significant effects when used in conjunction with other weight-loss compounds. Two good published studies found no consistent results. In a study by Usiskin and colleagues, no changes in body composition were demonstrated, even at 1,600 mg per day in obese men. Normal-weight men showed reduced body fat only for a brief time. A longer study by Morales and colleagues found no changes of significance in either men or women over a period of three months while using replacement levels of DHEA. Nevertheless, and although there are many individual exceptions, women who have the highest circulating levels of DHEA generally have the lowest body-mass indexes.[75]

Additionally, benefits have been reported for bodybuilders and others who would like to increase lean tissue and reduce body fat with DHEA. In 1995, at the New York Academy of Science's Conference on DHEA, D. Jakubowicz and colleagues of Venezuela, reported their results in a trial in which 300 mg of DHEA was given nightly for one month to twenty-two men, ages fifty-five to fifty-nine. Insulin levels fell 27 percent, insulin-like growth factor (IGF-1) increased 89 percent, body fat fell 14 percent, and lean tissue increased 7.8 percent. In the general discussion that closed the conference, Dr. Jorge Flechas maintained that although most people do not lose weight with DHEA, they do feel better and more vital, and men see a drop in LDL cholesterol and total cholesterol levels.

There are four ways in which DHEA may improve the lean-to-fat ratio of the body. These include influencing insulin levels and response, reducing food intake, reducing fat intake, and increasing thermogenesis. A potential fifth mechanism is DHEA's effect upon cortisol levels in the body. The first point is easy to document. DHEA levels are often inversely correlated with those of insulin, and this may be a reason why some individuals lose weight when they take the hormone. DHEA has been shown to increase the sensitivity of cells to insulin in humans.

Anecdotal reports indicate that DHEA reduces food intake in humans. Unfortunately, the only real studies have been conducted with animals, specifically, with rats genetically bred to become obese (Zucker strain). The inclusion of high doses of DHEA in the diets of these animals resulted in reductions in the amount of fat and protein that the animals voluntarily ate. After DHEA was removed from the diet, in at least one of the studies, the animals experienced rebound eating. Again, the implications for humans are not clear.

DHEA may increase thermogenesis by altering energy production in the liver. Most thermogenic compounds are either beta-adrenergic agonists (that is, increase the stimulation of beta-receptors) or are alpha-adrenergic antagonists (hence, reduce the activation of alpha-receptors). DHEA, however, appears to direct glucose utilization into an energy production pathway. This would account for at least some of the mood elevation and feelings of greater energy that are routinely reported with the use of DHEA. It also suggests once again that DHEA may be significant for weight loss only as part of a synergistic combination of compounds.

Finally, cortisol production provides an interesting marker for aging in that its secretion is inversely correlated with DHEA production. The ability to keep the synthesis of these hormones in balance and yet meet daily needs is called an *adaptive response,* or the *stress response.* Most of the adaptive responses of the body decline markedly with age and with chronic stress; it is clear that aging and disturbances within the body's adaptive stress response are closely linked. This connection has been explored by a number of researchers, among them Hans Selye. The stress response involves a feedback loop that links production of corticotropin-releasing hormone (CRH) provided by the hypothalamus, to that of adrenocorticotropic hormone (ACTH) found in the pituitary gland, to the release of corticosteroid hormones, such as cortisol, by the adrenal gland. Frequent and uncontrolled stress depletes DHEA levels—production is limited by the rate at which cholesterol is converted into DHEA—and disturbs the overall feedback mechanism between the adrenal cortex and the hypothalamus. Excessive cortisol production also causes a series of alterations in the general nature of the metabolism, again making a return to homeostasis more and more difficult. Elevated cortisol levels, of course, lead to the loss of lean tissues and, ultimately, to weight gain in many individuals.

7-keto-DHEA appears to have a thermogenic effect in the body that is mediated via the liver. Moreover, at least in animals, 7-oxo-DHEA (that is, 7-keto-DHEA) is more effective than DHEA as an inducer of liver mitochondrial activity. It has been suggested that 7-keto-DHEA induces a proton or "energy leak" in the mitochondrial membrane. A similar "leak" has been demonstrated as part of the thermogenic action of the active thyroid hormone known as T3.[76] Unfortunately, there do not appear to be any published peer-reviewed journal articles dealing with clinical weight-loss trials using 7-keto-DHEA.

Other Benefits of DHEA[77]

- Improves the symptoms of rheumatoid arthritis.
- May be a chemopreventative agent against cancer.[78]
- May prevent or reverse some forms of diabetes.
- Enhances the functions of the immune system.
- Improves brain function.
- Protects against infections.
- May be a substitute for estrogen replacement.
- Exhibits life-extension properties in laboratory animals.

Availability and Usage

It is sometimes claimed that DHEA is found in Mexican wild yam, but most herbalists consider the Mexican yam to contain a pro-steroid compound that cannot be manipulated by human physiology to produce DHEA. However, this pro-steroid can be synthetically altered to produce DHEA.

In a Stanford University study, a dose of 50 mg of DHEA given at bedtime to men and women, aged forty to seventy, restored them to early-adult blood levels within two weeks. Some researchers maintain that DHEA is metabolized in the body within eight hours. This suggests that taking divided doses of 25 mg in the morning and in the evening (best taken before meals) would be a preferred regimen. There is no consensus available on dosage levels, other than that women should use only roughly half the dosage used by men because of size differences and because DHEA has very mild androgenic effects. In a lupus study utilizing 200 mg of DHEA per day, half the women reported acne, and some reported increased facial hair. In a similar study performed at Stanford University and published in 1994, a few women developed facial hair, even on dosages of 100 mg. According to many published reports, supplementation with 200 mg of DHEA per day leads to acne or hirsutism (excessive growth of hair) in about 40 percent of women patients treated. However, many doctors report routinely giving older women 50 mg per day without side effects.

The majority of researchers consider DHEA supplementation to be inadvisable for men and (especially) women below the age of forty-five unless there are special reasons for its use. Dosages should be 10–50 mg per day *for women*, depending upon age and other factors. *For men, dosages should be between 25 and 100 mg per day. Dosages above these levels may cause androgenic effects in women and estrogenic effects in men.* Some doctors who specialize in sports medicine have reported that body-builders using very high dosages of DHEA for extended periods of time have exhibited signs of elevated estrogen levels. Inasmuch as sex hormone production is closely regulated by the body, with each sex's primary pathway being the most closely regulated, it is possible to upregulate the alternate pathway.

The most promising area of potential benefit of DHEA for dieters is in a synergistic combination with other diet aids. Some studies have shown, for instance, that DHEA improves the efficacy of the diet drug fenfluramine when the two compounds are taken together. It is known that the brain, including the special region of the hypothalamus that regulates appetite, has receptors for DHEA and/or DHEA metabolites. Fen-fluramine alters levels of the brain chemical serotonin and specifically involves the hypothalamus. This suggests that DHEA may influence satiety in conjunction with the same mechanisms. Therefore, DHEA may improve the effects of compounds that influence appetite and energy levels, even though DHEA itself, when used alone, has only a mild effect upon body weight. For other benefits found with DHEA, the reader is advised to consult *The ABC's of Hormones* by Jack Challem (McGraw-Hill/Contemporary Books, 1999). Those interested in supplementing with anything above small amounts of DHEA, that is, above 5–10 mg per day, should consult a physician and have blood levels of DHEA-S measured.

As an aid to weight loss, individuals might try 100–200 mg of 7-keto-DHEA (in divided doses) for one or two months. If supplementing with 7-keto-DHEA beyond this length of time, again, it would be a good idea to consult a physician.

Caution

Men with enlarged prostates or prostatic cancer and women with reproductive cancers, breast cancer, or endometriosis should avoid DHEA. These conditions, which are stimulated by androgens and estrogens, may be stimulated by the androgenic aspects of DHEA. However, there is no consensus to date regarding the effects of DHEA upon sex-hormone-sensitive cancers.

DIGESTIVE AIDS (PANCREATIN, BROMELAIN, PAPAIN, AND OTHERS)

From the moment food enters the mouth, it is attacked by a variety of digestive enzymes. Enzymes are proteins that serve as catalysts for the breakdown of food components. Saliva contains *amylase,* which begins the digestion of starches. In the stomach, both hydrochloric acid and the enzyme *pepsin* digest proteins. The pancreas is an organ that not only provides insulin to control blood sugar levels, but also produces amylase to split starches into more simple sugars, other proteases (protein-digesting enzymes) to further break down proteins, and the enzyme *lipase* to digest fats. The liver, the gallbladder, and the intestinal wall itself supply yet other digestive enzymes. The rather complex mixture of digestive elements secreted by the pancreas is commonly lumped under the single heading *pancreatin,* which is the defatted and dried powder of raw pancreatic enzymes.

A number of plant, yeast, fungal, and bacterial substances can serve to improve the digestion of various components of the diet. Bromelain, which is found in raw pineapple, and papain, which comes from papaya, are powerful protein-digesting substances. The culture of *Aspergillus* (a fungus) is used similarly as the source of many active enzymes, including forms of protease, amylase, lipase, cellulase, and lactase.

It should be noted that many people whose digestive systems are underactive may have acquired *Candida albicans* (yeast) infections, or otherwise lack the proper intestinal flora. Yeast infections are difficult to prove, but they are suspected in many cases of unexplained fatigue, water retention, weight gain, immune suppression, and allergies. A number of products attempt to correct these conditions by killing the offending yeast and by supplementing the normal intestinal flora with bacteria that are known to be found in the healthy gastrointestinal tract. For more on this, see the discussion "Other Digestive Issues" on page 40.

How Digestive Aids Help with Weight Loss

Since many diet products claim to work by interfering with the digestion or absorption of fats, it may seem strange that digestive aids can help you lose weight. However, evidence points in this direction. In animal experiments, supplementation with pancreatin both reduced food intake and led to weight loss. Why this should be the case is not entirely clear. Sometimes weight gain is triggered as a response to the body's perceived lack of calories or nutrients. In such instances the weight gain may be reversed following the improved digestion that comes with the use of pancreatin. The role of nutrition in shunting calories into the lean tissues and into activity will be discussed in Chapter 5. No matter what one's weight may be, impaired digestion, malabsorption, and nutritional deficiencies will lead to ill health. In those who are overweight, the symptoms will disproportionately be those of lowered thyroid activity, sluggishness, fluid retention, inflammation, and the like. Having said this, we nevertheless should point out that digestive enzymes are, at best, mild aids to weight loss and likely will have a significant effect upon weight only when used in conjunction with other, more powerful diet aids.

Bromelain, which is primarily involved in the digestion of protein, is more narrow in its effects than is pancreatin. For best results, bromelain should be combined with pancreatin and bile. Papain, which is derived from the unripe papaya, not only digests protein but wheat gluten as well. This is quite a bonus, for difficulty in digesting gluten is quite common.

Animal sources of digestive aids tend to be stronger and more broad-spectrum than plant and bacterial sources, with pork-derived pancreatin being much stronger than that from oxen.

Other Benefits of Digestive Aids[79]

- Pancreatin and bromelain have been shown to improve the body's response to inflammation and swelling, and therefore to be useful for diseases such as rheumatoid arthritis. Used in conjunction, bromelain improves the absorption of pancreatin.

- Proteolytic (protein-digesting) enzymes help prevent and remove fibrin clots in blood and lymph vessels.

- Proteases improve the body's ability to remove circulating immune complexes (byproducts of immune system activities) from the blood and thus protect the kidneys and improve immune responses while reducing autoimmune reactions.

- By preventing undigested protein from reaching the small intestine, pancreatin and other protein-digesting enzymes may serve to reduce allergies, food sensitivities, and a host of other reactions to foreign proteins that reach the bloodstream.

- Bromelain may block the production of the prostaglandins that make the blood "sticky."

- Bromelain and other proteolytic enzymes improve the body's ability to turn over the protein content of the tissues, and thus they help in the healing of soft tissue injuries, such as those often encountered in sports.

- Bromelain may improve the absorption of antibiotics, antioxidants, and other compounds into the tissues.[80]

Availability and Usage

Pancreatin is sold in terms of its activity or strength, not its weight. If the pancreatin is listed as 4X USP, for instance, the dosage might be 2–4 tablets with meals; at 8X or 10X the dosage would be 1 or 2 tablets. Another unit used is NF (natural formulary), which is of a similar potency to the U.S.P. (U.S. Pharmacopeia). Since many standards are used, there is some confusion over equivalencies among products. Pancreatin, bromelain, and papain are often combined with betaine HCl (betaine hydrochloric acid) to improve digestion in the stomach. Formulas may contain a number of enzymes mixed together, for example, amylase, protease, lipase, and cellulase may be combined, or these may be added to a formula based upon pancreatin. Always start with a conservative dosage, work up to a satisfactory amount, and cut back the dosage as your digestive ability improves.

Bromelain and papain are sold by weight in milligrams (mg) and by potencies. The common units of activity are MCU (milk-clotting units) and GDU (gelatin-digesting units). For a potency of 2,000 GDU, you would use 250–500 mg of bromelain with meals, or 500–1,000 mg of papain. Many studies recommend 2,000–4,000 mg of bromelain a day! For inflammation and other such special uses, these two enzymes are taken between meals rather than with them. However, those with ulcers or similar gastrointestinal problems should consult their doctors before trying such dosages.

Most of the quality research conducted to assess the health benefits of digestive enzymes has been performed in Europe using the brand-name product Wobenzyme.

As a final note, there are herbal "bitters" (usually based upon extracts of *Gentiana lutea*) and other herbal digestive stimulants on the market. Some bitters are actually used as flavorings for drinks and in cooking.

Other Digestive Issues

Faulty carbohydrate metabolism is sometimes linked to intestinal invasion by the yeast *Candida albicans.* Those suspecting this problem should consult specialized literature, such as Scott J. Gregory's *A Holistic Protocol for the Immune System* (Tree of Life Publications, 1989) and Luc De Schepper's *Candida* (LDS Publications, 1986) and *Peak Immunity* (Le Fever, 1989). Approaches to controlling yeast overgrowth include killing the yeast with products such as nystatin, citrus extract, or other anti-yeast substances, and supplementing with *Lactobacillus acidophilus,* the much hardier bacteria *S. faecium 68,* and other beneficial organisms. Beneficial bacterial products are available through many different companies. As a rule, success in implanting friendly bacteria, such as *L. acidophilus,* in the face of a yeast overgrowth often requires the prior use of an anti-yeast product. A specialty bacterial strain, *Bacillus laterosporus* (BOD strain), is recommended by Gregory, De Schepper, and some candida support groups for its anti-yeast benefits. Although considered effective for this purpose, *B. laterosporus* is presently the subject of considerable controversy. It is sometimes contained in formulations listing "soil-based organisms."

FAT BLOCKERS. STARCH BLOCKERS. AND FAT AND SUGAR SUBSTITUTES

A natural way to reduce the body's absorption of fat and sugar is to increase the consumption of fiber, especially from vegetables. Commercial sugar substitutes that provide the sweet flavor without the calories have been around for a long time. New products have now appeared that work specifically to reduce the absorption of fat or to replace the fats usually found in foods. In the category of fat blockers, the primary products are made from a type of fiber called chitosan, which directly binds fats before they can be absorbed, and a protein fraction (a peptide) that both binds to fats and increases their clearance from the digestive tract. In the second category, fat substitutes, we find the product Olean (olestra). All of these approaches to reducing caloric intake claim to help dieters.

Chitosan is an extract from the hard outer shells, or exoskeletons, of shellfish. In Japan this type of material was developed for purification of water and other substances, especially in the food industry. The principle is that there is a positive electrical charge on the chitosan, which draws oppositely charged materials to it. The same type of fiber was developed in Europe, where the principle of electrical charge was recognized as having a bearing on fat absorption. Fats and bile acids are negatively charged, and therefore are attracted to the chitosan, which binds them before they can enter the bloodstream. The makers of chitosan products claim that fats equal to seven to eight times the weight of the chitosan can be blocked and eliminated from the body in this fashion.

A quite different approach to absorbing and trapping fats uses components found in certain proteins. What is called "globin digest" is prepared by a special acidic protease (protein-digesting) treatment. Peptide FM is the brand name for the small chain of peptides that makes up globin digest. A combination of bovine (cow) milk and/or wheat proteins provide the starting materials. The claim is that the digestion, absorption, and metabolism of fats are regulated by this material. Another peptide that is said to influence appetite is glycomacropeptide (bovine kappa-caseino glycomacropeptide, or GMP) from whey protein.

Yet another protein is the key ingredient in Starch Blocker. Starch Blocker received a great deal of attention a few years ago. The FDA once ordered it to be removed from the marketplace, although it is now again being sold with somewhat more limited claims. Starch Blocker contains the protein *phaseolamine,* a compound that interferes with the digestion of starch. Phaseolamine is an extract of the bean *Phaseolus vulgaris.*

No true "sugar blocker" is available. However, non-digestible sugar substitutes, whether sugar alcohols or specially altered amino acids, such as those that make up aspartame (NutraSweet), have been around long enough to become part of billion-dollar industries. If we can have faux sugar, why not faux fat? Olestra is a "fat-free fat" marketed as Olean by Procter & Gamble (developed at a cost reputedly well above 200 million dollars). The basic principle is simple: Regular fat consists of fatty acids arranged around a type of alcohol called glycerol. In the digestive tract, various enzymes cut through the intestinal wall and into the blood. Olestra, however, has a very large center made of sucrose (sugar) instead of glycerol, and around this center are arranged six to eight fatty acids. The result is a molecule that is much bigger than normal fats and that has fatty acids so tightly packed together that digestive enzymes cannot reach the crucial links to snip off the fatty-acid components. The olestra molecule itself is too massive to pass through the intestinal wall.

The health food industry, for better or worse, has attempted to copy the olestra approach to weight loss. There is now available a lipase inhibitor (blocker of fat digestion) derived from *Cassia nomame mimosoides.* Clearly, this item was developed to mimic the actions of the pharmaceutical weight-loss product called Xenical (orlistat), which inhibits the absorption of 30 percent of fat found in the diet. Not addressed in the advertisements is whether the side effects of the pharmaceutical drug are also found. No direct trials have been performed to prove that this item works as well as the pharmaceutical compound.

How Do They Work?

Chitosan has been tested more than once against the FDA-approved drug Questran (cholestyramine). Questran removes bile acids from the liver and effectively lowers cholesterol levels. Chitosan binds liver bile acids, but it primarily binds dietary cholesterol and other fats. In head-to-head tests, the drug was more effective at lowering cholesterol, yet the researchers were able to conclude, "chitosan may have lipid-lowering effects similar to those of cholestyramine."[81] Chitosan is used to reduce the body's absorption of fat from the diet. In effect, it is intended to allow the dieter to follow a low-fat diet without cutting fat from the diet.

The European supplier of chitosan reported that weight-loss results for people who took the extract were twice those found with the controls during the first two weeks, and roughly another 5 pounds better over the next two weeks. Blood-pressure-lowering effects were also significant. Compared to Questran, chitosan is certainly safe.[82] Nevertheless, some researchers have questioned the wisdom of long-term use of chitosan.

The original use of this type of fiber in Japan was to clear metals from water, and, as this implies, chitosan may bind minerals found in the diet as well as fats. Similarly, chitosan is unlikely to distinguish between fat-soluble vitamins and other such nutrients; therefore, a deficiency in vitamins such as A and E and in nutrients such as beta-carotene might develop. Japanese researchers have actually performed experiments with animals to see if chitosan taken in large amounts will have a negative effect on the mineral and vitamin status of the body. They found that mineral absorption was greatly decreased, the bones were demineralized, and there was a "marked and rapid decrease in the serum vitamin E level."[83]

More generally, a cynic might point out that chitosan, to be effective, must be used in amounts similar to those that are effective with plant-fiber sources. This is to say that although chitosan may have weight-loss benefits if ingested in adequate amounts, these benefits are not striking for what is, in effect, a fiber substitute.

Phaseolamine (Starch Blocker) works by inhibiting the actions of alpha-amylase, an enzyme produced by the pancreas and released into the small intestine. When taken in sufficient amounts, phaseolamine can block the digestion of a significant quantity of ingested starch.[84] The benefit is not only a reduction in the calories absorbed, but also a reduction in the amount of sugar absorbed inasmuch as all starches are ultimately absorbed as glucose. Phaseolamine, therefore, is an aid to dieters and other individuals who desire to reduce their absorption of carbohydrates and to shift the diet's effective energy ratio away from sugars and toward other energy sources, such as protein.[85]

Carbohydrates come in three forms: The non-digestible types are called fibers. Digestible carbohydrates are either complex—a category made up primarily of starches—or simple, which is to say, sugars. Most individuals now realize that the excessive consumption of sugars is bad for health; nevertheless, an elevated consumption of sugars is very hard to avoid in modern, processed diets. Complex carbohydrates, including starches, are universally converted to glucose (sugar) before being absorbed. Starch is found primarily in grains (breads, pastas, cereals, rice) and also in potatoes, corn, and a number of other foods. Not only do these starches ultimately end up as glucose, in the highly refined forms we normally consume, but they do so very quickly. In conjunction with the sugars already found in the modern diet, this presents a definite problem for carbohydrate metabolism. Phaseolamine, used appropriately, can inhibit digestion and delay the absorption of several hundred calories derived from starches.

In several unpublished studies, Peptide FM (globin digest) was shown to decrease total body fat and serum triglycerides in humans as well as in animals. Over a three-month period, body-fat levels typically were reduced about 3 percent with no other changes in diet or exercise. The explanation offered by researchers is that movement of fat into the bloodstream from ingested food is reduced and that the overall turnover of fats by the body, including oxidation for energy, is increased.[86] A further claim that the synthesis of new fat from carbohydrates is reduced is probably an indirect effect of the improved insulin response that is usually found when there is better clearance of free fatty acids from the blood. No side effects have been reported.

GMP is a more interesting compound. The biological activity of GMP has received much attention, with research focused on the ability of GMP to bind cholera and *Escherichia coli* enterotoxins, inhibit bacterial and viral adhesion, suppress gastric secretions, promote bifidobacterial growth, and modulate immune system responses. Protection against toxins, bacteria, and viruses, and modulation of the immune system are considered to be the most promising applications.[87] Some have suggested that GMP may influence gastric emptying via an effect upon cholecystokinin (CCK), mentioned earlier under APPETITE SUPPRESSANTS on page 12.[88] Whether GMP has any special weight-loss benefits has yet to be demonstrated.

Olestra, the nonfat fat, is included here because soon it will be found routinely in the food chain, from chips and dips to ice cream and beyond. It works by simply replacing fats in the diet with a non-digestible sucrose polymer. Unfortunately, various researchers, including those who testified before the FDA, have noted that olestra binds and removes fat-soluble nutrients from the body. This includes carotenes and vitamins A, D, F, and K. Olestra also apparently causes diarrhea in some individuals.[89]

An interesting secondary issue is whether these calorie-free sweeteners and fats succeed in helping dieters lose weight. More than one bariatrician (a doctor who specializes in obesity) has told the authors that dieters who do not lose weight when treated medically typically are those who drink the largest amounts of sugar-free diet drinks. This curious result could come from the amount of sodium found in those drinks, which might encourage water retention in some individuals, or other factors might be involved. Saccharin may in fact help slightly with weight loss under some conditions, but aspartame appears to downregulate the enzyme responsible for thermogenesis by as much as 30 percent! In either case, however, the mere use of artificial sweeteners may lead to greatly increased fat consumption when compared with a similar use of sugar. Similarly, one study found that when subjects consumed artificially sweetened drinks during exercise, they ate 160–190 more calories from all sources at lunch than did individuals who drank plain water or a sucrose-flavored drink![90]

One likely explanation is that the mere "sweet taste" on the tongue may stimulate the release of insulin. Research on this point has been equivocal for the moderate consumption of "sweet taste" (which does not rule out the suggestion). In contrast, it does seem to be clearly proven that the consumption of "sham" foods that taste like the real thing, but which have no calories, leads to significant elevations of blood insulin levels. When olestra was used to replace fat calories in a restricted-calorie diet, a recent study found that dieters simply ate more calories to make up for the lost fat calories if given access to more food.[91] *The implication is that the consumption of the new reduced-calorie imitation foods will not help dieters either take off or keep off weight.*

Availability and Usage

Chitosan is taken in amounts that vary to match the fat content of a meal. It is available in tablets and capsules. Directions come with the products; for example, one slice of pizza with 20 grams of fat might be balanced with 10 chitosan capsules. Peptide FM will usually be found as a component in diet powders and similar products. The amount recommended to control the fat in an average diet is between 1.5 and 2 grams. However, extrapolations from what data we have would suggest that intakes of up to 4 grams may be required. Relatively large doses may also be required with phaseolamine if this substance is to be used for maintaining what is effectively a low-carbohydrate diet—even when carbohydrates are being ingested. One or two grams per meal of this active ingredient may be required, so manufacturers directions must be followed closely.

FIBER

Fiber exists in soluble, semi-soluble, and insoluble forms. Insoluble fibers are those for which humans lack digestive enzymes, and which therefore do not break down significantly in the digestive tract. Cellulose from grain brans, some parts of fruits and vegetables, and lignin from legumes are insoluble fibers. These fibers provide roughage to ensure bowel movements.

Soluble fibers, which do break down under the action of our digestive enzymes, include pectins and gums (mucilages). About a third of the fiber in fruits, vegetables, and many legumes is soluble. Some grains, such as oats and barley, contain large amounts of soluble fibers. These are considered highly desirable fibers. Pectins have long been known to promote wound healing, to slow the absorption of glucose from the intestines into the bloodstream, to bind a number of toxic chemicals, thus preventing their absorption, and to aid in the reduction of cholesterol levels through the binding of bile acids.[92]

Hemicellulose has qualities of both insoluble and soluble fibers. Psyllium husks, the dried seed coat of *Plantago ovata*, is perhaps the best of these. It acts as roughage and absorbs and removes toxins from the intestines. It also moistens and soothes irritated intestinal membranes.

How Fiber Helps with Weight Loss

It is now recognized that the addition of fiber to the diet, especially soluble and semi-soluble fibers, offers many health benefits. Mixtures of fibers of various types can be designed to work together synergistically to maximize their health-promoting properties. They act to regularize bowel functions, including the control of both diarrhea and constipation, to soothe irritated mucous membranes in the gastrointestinal tract, and to absorb various toxins and bacteria, which are then eliminated with the help of the bulking action of the fibers. Psyllium husks have long been used in traditional medical systems, such as that of the Ayurvedic tradition, to perform precisely these functions.[93] As already noted, they have properties of both soluble and non-soluble fibers, but do not produce the gas and bloating nor the intestinal irritation characteristic of crude fibers, such as wheat bran.[94]

Emphasis upon the role of fiber in weight loss has once again become a topic of interest at the beginning of the twenty-first century because of the relative failure of reduced-fat diets to produce the hoped-for results. As one review puts it, "the previous focus on lowering dietary fat as a means for promoting negative energy balance has led to an underestimation of the potential role of dietary composition in promoting reductions in energy intake and weight loss."[95] Fiber plays an important role in helping to reduce excess weight. The bulk of the fiber itself gives a physical sensation of fullness that helps to control how much is eaten at a given meal. Appetite is reduced directly by the bulk of the fiber and indirectly through the delayed emptying of the stomach and the release of brain and gastrointestinal-tract hormones that signal satiety.[96]

The bulking action of soluble fibers significantly slows the release of carbohydrates into the blood from the intestines. The limited post-meal rise in blood sugar levels associated with the consumption of complex carbohydrates, especially with those of vegetables and legumes, likewise moderates the release of insulin into the blood and avoids both the health dangers and the surges in appetite that characterize the body's responses to excessive insulin release.[97] Some have suggested that adding fiber to meals can help reduce the impact of carbohydrates on the glycemic response.[98]

Just how important is dietary fiber in controlling weight? One study found that lean individuals eat about 50 percent more fiber than do those who are either moderately or severely obese. The amount of fiber in the diets of the three groups was estimated to be 18.8 grams in lean individuals, 13.3 grams in moderately obese individuals, and 13.7 grams in severly obese individuals. Other significant roles for fiber include the lowering of total cholesterol and the reduction of the incidence of colorectal cancer. People who consume the most fiber have 47 percent less colorectal cancer and 66 percent less pancreatic cancer than those who eat the least fiber.[99] Since colon cancer ranks just behind lung cancer as a cause of death, the protection afforded by fiber against this particular cancer is of considerable importance.[100]

Availability and Usage

The preferred sources of fiber are the soluble and semi-soluble varieties. Pectin, guar gum, oat bran, barley, and psyllium seed husks are such sources. Some of the new fiber products made from citrus sources may also come under this heading of preferred fibers. Whole foods can supply significant amounts of fiber. Oats, barley, oat bran, and various legumes can be added to the diet on a regular basis to supply sufficient quantities of these fiber groups. However, if this is not possible, the more concentrated of these fibers are available in tablets, capsules, and powdered or granulated forms. Two to four tablets or capsules, or 1 to 2 teaspoons of granules or powder, can be taken an hour before meals. These dosages should always be taken with at least 8 or more ounces of water so that serious dehydration does not result.

Caution

Although most of us can probably benefit from adding fiber to our diets, too much of a good thing, including fiber, can create problems. This is especially true of the insoluble fibers such as wheat bran. Fiber also can be hard on the intestines if taken in excess. Some symptoms of excess fiber consumption are bloating, diarrhea, and nausea. Moreover, just as fiber can absorb toxins from the colon, most types of fiber can interfere with the absorption of some nutrients. Therefore, it may be a good idea to take fiber supplements at a different time than when you take your meals or your vitamin and mineral supplements.

GAMMA-LINOLENIC ACID (GLA), FLAX, AND THE OMEGA-3 ESSENTIAL FATTY ACIDS

With the current constant push to reduce the intake of fats in the diet, it is easy to forget that certain fats are essential for health and that other fats, although not essential, are powerful health promoters. The essential fatty acids (EFAs) must be supplied by the diet. These and other fats are required for the absorption of fat-soluble vitamins and related nutrients. The EFAs also make up significant portions of the nervous tissue in the brain and elsewhere, and are building blocks for the body's production of hormones (including the sterol hormones testosterone and estrogen) and hormonelike signaling compounds (such as prostaglandins). The two families of EFAs are the omega-6 family, which is based upon linoleic acid (LA), and the omega-3 family, which is based upon alpha-linolenic acid (LNA). These are discussed in turn.

Gamma-linolenic acid (GLA) is an omega-6 fatty-acid nutrient. Under ideal circumstances, it is made in the body from the conversion of linoleic acid. GLA serves as a precursor to the family of hormonelike substances or "activated fatty acids" known as PGE-1, meaning the prostaglandin (PG) family "E" derived from GLA. The PGE-1 family is involved in anti-inflammatory, anti-spasm, anti-infection, and similar actions in the body, including reducing the "stickiness" of the blood.

A second family of prostaglandins, PGE-2, is made from the omega-6 linoleic acid through an intermediate step that creates arachidonic acid; it is also made directly from the arachidonic acid readily found in the American diet. This PGE-2 series activates aspects of the immune system as well as other systems, but in excess it leads to inflammation, menstrual cramps, asthma, heart disease, and many other problems including, in some cases, obesity. Among its other duties, the PGE-1 family serves to control or to turn off the PGE-2 family.

Many factors can prevent the conversion of linoleic acid to GLA, and GLA to PGE-1. These factors include deficiencies of the vitamins B_3, B_6, C, and biotin, as well as deficiencies in the minerals magnesium and zinc. Too much alcohol, too much saturated fat, the consumption of hydrogenated oils (*trans*-fatty acids) and heat-damaged fats, and many other dietary factors may contribute to the body's inability to perform this conversion. Moreover, many people (especially those who tend to put on weight) have difficulty transforming linoleic acid into GLA simply because they naturally produce relatively little of the enzyme needed for this transformation.[101]

The omega-3 fatty acid alpha-linolenic acid is found abundantly in flaxseed oil, whereas docoshexaenoic acid (DHA) and eicosapentaenoic acid (EPA) are found primarily in cold-water ocean fish, such as salmon and sardines. Although they are closely related fatty acids, EPA and DHA have somewhat different effects within the body. EPA exerts its major activity by suppressing the arachidonic acid cascade and by increasing the production of anti-inflammatory prostaglandins, in particular the family of prostaglandins called PGE-3. DHA has a larger repertoire of uses in the body. For instance, it acts as a ready source of EPA because it can be reconverted to EPA when needed. However, DHA is far more than merely a potential source of EPA. DHA is critical for the proper functioning of the nervous system. It also has a stronger effect upon levels of blood lipids.[102] Although EPA can be converted to DHA, the rate of conversion may be inadequate to meet periods of chronic and/or elevated demand, and therefore supplemental DHA, and not just LNA and/or EPA, may be of importance for maintaining normal health. As with GLA, the transformation of these fatty acids—from LNA to EPA to DHA and then to their active PGE-3 prostaglandins—can be blocked by diets low in minerals and high in *trans*-fatty acids. Hence, although flaxseed oil as a supplier of LNA may be the least expensive source of omega-3 fatty acids, individuals who need therapeutic levels of supplementation should strongly consider using concentrated sources of EPA and DHA.

There is considerable agreement that for most of human history, and certainly before the advent of cereal grains, the ratio of omega-6 to omega-3 fatty acids in the diet was 2:1, or perhaps 3:1. In modern diets, the ratio is at least 10:1 and perhaps even as high as 20:1. Excessive intake of LA, especially in diets rich in refined carbohydrates, promotes heart disease, inflammation, and autoimmune disorders. Modern diets tend toward odd nutrient imbalances: They are high in *trans*-fatty acids and too high in LA. They are high in refined carbohydrates and rich in preformed arachidonic acid, but low in minerals and omega-3 fatty acids. As a result, the pathways to the anti-inflammatory and thyroid-supporting prostaglandins are either underfed or blocked.

How Essential Fatty Acids Can Help You Lose Fat

A study conducted in 1979 illustrates the effectiveness of GLA as a nutrient that promotes weight loss. In this study, thirty-eight individuals took GLA in the form of evening primrose oil for eight weeks. Of the subjects who were more than 10 percent above their ideal weights, half lost an average of 9 pounds while taking 4 capsules per day. Only five individuals in the group showed no weight change, and the four subjects who took 8 capsules per day averaged a weight loss of 23 pounds. One explanation for the effectiveness of GLA is that it appears to increase the level of brown fat NA/K ATPase activity. Brown fat (also called brown adipose tissue) readily burns fat stores for energy, and this specific enzyme (NA/K ATPase) controls the rate of metabolism.[103]

GLA and similarly active products are available in various forms, but it should be emphasized that essential fatty acids are foods, and the best approach is to correct the diet even if you plan to supplement. Many factors in the diet impede the absorption of EFAs. The most important of these factors are the consumption of refined and overheated vegetable oils; the presence in the diet of margarines and other sources of hydrogenated oils, which contain *trans*-fatty acids that produce negative effects in the body—

no, margarine is not good for you; and the consumption of too much saturated fat. Natural fats from unprocessed foods are almost entirely *cis*-fatty acids, which are of benefit to the body, and only rarely *trans*-fatty acids.

Frying with *any* polyunsaturated oil, such as peanut or cottonseed oil, damages that oil and impedes the absorption of EFAs contained both in those oils and in the foods cooked in them. Although it has a relatively low smoking point, olive oil, which is mostly monosaturated, is probably the best choice as an oil for frying. Frying with highly unsaturated oils is so unhealthful that even the much maligned animal fats may be preferable to, say, safflower, corn, or other such oils, for this task. *Trans*-fatty acids have long been known to adversely affect the immune system, to increase free-radical production, to produce abnormal sperm, to lower testosterone levels, and to impair the processing of insulin.[104]

Direct sources of GLA are expensive and difficult to keep fresh, although there are some excellent sources available. Your body can manufacture its own GLA from *cis*-linoleic acid, which can be found in unrefined, *cold-pressed* polyunsaturated vegetable oils. (These oils must be *cold-pressed* only. If they are not specifically labeled as such, they should be avoided.)

For those who are over their ideal weights, it may be best to assume that the body's ability to create GLA may be impaired. Thus, sources of pure GLA may be necessary. An alternative to supplementation with GLA is to supply alpha-linolenic acid. As indicated previously, this fatty acid can be used to create the PGE-3 family of prostaglandins, and the PGE-3s can perform most of the roles of the PGE-1s. Fish oils provide the precursors to PGE-3 and may be required in cases in which the omega-3 transformation pathways are operating poorly. Good plant sources of omega-3 fatty acids are rare, but they do exist and might be tried. As noted already, the richest plant source of LNA is fresh flaxseed oil. (Flaxseed oil always should be taken with a small amount of vitamin B_6, and it is best utilized when eaten with a bit of sulfur-containing protein, such as low-fat cottage cheese.)

More commonly available plant sources of LNA are pumpkin seed oil (15 percent), soy oil (9 percent, but so high in LA as to not be a recommended source of LNA), and walnut oil (5 percent). Again, these should be cold pressed and protected from heat and light. Fresh, raw pumpkin seeds and walnuts can be used in place of the oils. A tablespoon of one of these cold-pressed, unrefined oils twice a day should be sufficient.

Benefits of GLA and Omega-3 Fatty Acids[105]

- GLA is noted for its usefulness in relieving premenstrual syndrome (PMS).

- GLA and omega-3 fatty acids have important anti-inflammatory properties.

- GLA helps to control rheumatoid arthritis. Omega-3 fatty acids also work to control arthritis and other similar degenerative conditions.

- Both GLA and omega-3 fatty acids have proven effective against cancer cells in vitro, and they are used abroad in some human cancer treatments.

- GLA and omega-3 fatty acids combat heart disease by lowering blood viscosity and by reducing LDL levels while decreasing blood platelet "stickiness." Omega-3 fatty acids raise HDL levels.

- Both GLA and omega-3 fatty acids combat high blood pressure.

- Both GLA and omega-3 fatty acids have shown usefulness in combating acne, eczema, and other skin problems.

- GLA and omega-3 fatty acids may help with prostate-gland problems.

- LNA has been shown to act as a substrate for the activities of various B vitamins. A deficiency of omega-3 fatty acids is implicated as a basic cause of depression and major mental illnesses. The PGE-3 family plays a role in regulating parts of the nervous system throughout the body.

- Both GLA and omega-3 fatty acids play roles in improving immune response.

- GLA has been shown to have benefits in cases of diabetic neuropathy (nerve damage). Over the course of a year, a large dose of GLA (480 mg daily) improved nerve status in thirteen out of sixteen measures in a controlled study.

- Omega-3 fatty acids appear to improve insulin sensitivity, to increase the oxidation of fats for fuel, to promote thermogenesis, and to help reduce fat storage. Unlike GLA, omega-3 fatty acids cannot serve as a substrate for the synthesis of arachidonic acid.

Availability and Usage

GLA appears to be more important for improving weight control than are the omega-3 fatty acids. It is found in significant amounts in human mother's milk, the seed oil of the evening primrose plant, borage oil, and black currant seed oil. Doses from 90 mg to as much as 400 mg of GLA have proven effective. This is the amount of GLA found in two to eight 500-mg capsules of evening primrose seed oil. Some individuals may find that they receive benefits only at the higher dosage range. GLA is often more effective when taken in conjunction with vitamin B_6 and vitamin E. Because in modern Western diets omega-3 fatty acids are almost always underrepresented and GLA (an omega-6 fatty acid) will do nothing to correct this imbalance, dieters should consider supplementing with 2–3 grams of high-potency/high-purity omega-3 fatty acids from fish oil each day (500 mg–1 gram with each meal) and/or adding flaxseed oil (1–2 tablespoons) to the diet. Ground or cracked flaxseed supplies lignans and other healthful ingredients, but it should not be consumed in amounts greater than 4 tablespoons per day due to the presence of tiny amounts of cyanogenic glycosides, substances which in excess have an unwanted impact upon thyroid hormone function.

GLA has been reported to give rise to occasional mild acne. In the experience of one clinical bariatrician, large doses given to improve weight loss also may lead to increased susceptibility to bruising in a small number of individuals. GLA and the omega-3 fatty acids are polyunsaturated fatty acids and therefore need protection against oxidation and free-radical damage. Concurrent daily usage of natural vitamin E (200–400 IU), grape seed extract polyphenols (100–300 mg), and/or alpha-lipoic acid (100–300 mg) is suggested. Concurrent intake of omega-3 fatty acids plus broad-spectrum antioxidant, and vitamin and mineral supplementation may help to prevent GLA from being transformed into arachidonic acid and the "bad" prostaglandins.

Individuals who are taking prescribed blood thinners should consult their doctors before adding these essential oils to the diet in any quantity. As indicated above, both GLA and the omega-3 fatty acids act as natural blood thinners and anticoagulants.

GRAPEFRUIT

Grapefruit has been used as a weight-loss aid for many years. This citrus fruit is high in pectin, a soluble fiber that lowers cholesterol and increases the amount of fat excreted from the body. Some studies involving pectin have shown that it markedly increases the amount of fat removed from the body. (See FIBER on page 46.) As a whole fruit, grapefruit provides vitamins, some minerals, considerable roughage, but very few calories. It also helps to correct the acid balance of the blood. As an aid to weight loss, it may deserve some of the reputation that it has. However, it does not work miracles. Grapefruit in pill form offers few benefits.

GROWTH HORMONE (GH) RELEASERS

Growth hormone releasers are amino acids and other compounds that can stimulate the pituitary gland's secretion of growth hormone (GH, also referred to as human growth hormone, or HGH). The most commonly suggested releasers are L-arginine, L-ornithine, L-tyrosine (better used as an appetite suppressant), L-tryptophan (banned by the FDA on questionable grounds), and L-glycine. Taken individually or in combination, these amino acids are reputed to raise the body's serum level of growth hormone. L-arginine and L-ornithine are the substances found in the nighttime weight-loss products that have been most highly advertised over the last few years.[107] The essential amino acid valine may prove to be more effective than either arginine or ornithine as a GH releaser when taken orally, but to date relatively little research has been performed with this amino acid.

Growth hormone is a natural hormone manufactured and stored in the pituitary gland. During our growing years, this hormone is responsible for the accelerated growth of our bones and muscles, for wound healing, for resistance to disease, and for the metabolism of fat stores. Unfortunately, the level of GH that is released declines gradually as we age, dropping rapidly after age thirty and becoming negligible after age fifty. The pituitary does not cease producing GH, but for reasons not well understood, the aging body gradually loses its ability to release the hormone. Obese individuals also seem less able to release GH, and obesity itself can play a causative role. The goal of GH-release programs is to raise the levels of GH release to those of adolescence or young adulthood.

Growth hormone is normally released one-half hour into sleep, during peak exercise, and in response to fasting or food deprivation. Vitamin B_6 is necessary for GH release, and supplemental choline and vitamin B_5 also may help. Evidence even points to a role for vitamin C, an important antioxidant.

A great deal of time and money has been expended by the pharmaceutical industry to produce orally active HGH secretagogues. The pharmaceutical company Merck & Co., Inc., recently stopped clinical trials of their oral growth-hormone booster, MK-0677, because it was not effective enough to bring to the market. Therefore, readers are urged to be very cautious regarding claims being made for supposedly effective HGH secretagogues that can be purchased in health food stores or even clinics when the major pharmaceutical companies have yet to market such products even as injectables. The remarks that follow are limited to much more restrained expectations, which might possibly ,be fulfilled in younger individuals through the proper use of nutrients.

How Do GH Releasers Work?

Growth hormone has many functions in the body. It stimulates protein production and collagen production, so it maintains and increases muscle tissue mass and it improves skin quality and the tone of the deeper layers of the dermis. More important for the dieter, GH causes fat stores to release fatty acids and forces them to be burned for energy.

The release of GH is controlled by two antagonistic hormones secreted by the hypothalamus gland of the brain. As its name suggests, the growth-hormone-releasing hormone (GHRH) causes the pituitary gland to release GH. The other hormone, somatostatin, turns off GH release. As we age, we become more sensitive to somatostatin and its inhibitory effects upon GH release. Aging slows down other aspects of GH release as well. For instance, aging diminishes the production of the neurotransmitter acetylcholine, thereby reducing the responsiveness to GHRH.

Furthermore, changes in insulin response are heavily implicated in the decline in responsiveness to GHRH and in the increase in sensitivity to somatostatin. GH release is usually triggered by low blood sugar levels, whereas somatostatin release is triggered by high blood sugar levels. Anything that upsets the insulin mechanism of the body therefore upsets GH release. Obesity, diets based upon simple carbohydrates, and diets lacking in chromium and other insulin-potentiating nutrients will all negatively affect GH release.[108]

Not all of the factors that cause declines in GH can be influenced, but certainly some can. The question is, How much? The usual supplements employed are L-arginine and L-ornithine, either alone or in combination. Most of the successful research results involved the injection of these amino acids, not their ingestion by mouth. Injection certainly produced dramatic results, but human tests with oral supplements often have shown only slight effects.[109] However, recent medical studies on burn and surgical patients have indicated that the alpha-ketoglutarate form of ornithine successfully maintains muscle mass and protein synthesis during severe trauma, which is to say, the effects of GH release.[110] GABA (gamma aminobutyric acid) is another special amino acid that appears to successfully cause the release of GH.[111]

Those suffering from seriously excessive weight gain tend not to respond well to GH releasers. Moreover, responsiveness to GH releasers declines in everyone after the age of thirty. The consensus is that we continue to produce adequate levels of GH, but that for some reason it is not released into the bloodstream as readily as during our younger years.

Other Benefits of GH Releasers

L-Arginine

- Stimulates the immune system.

- Promotes wound healing.

- Blocks the formation of tumors.

- Helps to regenerate the liver.

- Increases spermatogenesis (formation and development of sperm cells).

L-Ornithine

- Stimulates the immune system.

- Promotes wound healing.

- Scavenges free radicals.

- Helps to regenerate the liver.

Note: Excessive consumption of arginine or ornithine may activate arthritic symptoms and likewise activate a previously dormant herpes virus. Since these amino acids must exist in the body in a balance with the essential amino acid lysine, excessive consumption of their pure forms may create a lysine deficiency.

L-Tyrosine

- Helps to control depression and anxiety.

- Acts as an appetite suppressant.

- Acts as a mild antioxidant.

- Increases the production of melanin (skin pigment).

- Is a precursor to a thyroid hormone, as is L-phenylalanine.

L-Glycine

- Is effective for hyperacidity (often used as an antacid).

- Can be used as a food additive for its sweet taste.

- Is an important component of glutathione peroxidase, one of the body's antioxidant enzymes.

- May promote healing, especially when taken with arginine or ornithine.

GABA

- Lowers blood pressure and encourages sleep.

- Is considered to be an antistress, antianxiety nutrient.

L-GLUTAMINE[112]

L-glutamine deserves special consideration. It is discussed in the section on appetite suppressants in terms of its ability to help ward off weight gain on high-fat diets, but there is much more to the story. Although it is a nonessential amino acid, L-glutamine has become the focus of extensive scientific interest because of its important physiological role. Indeed, since the 1980s, many researchers have come to regard glutamine as "conditionally essential." Conditionally essential nutrients are those that the body can produce in quantities sufficient to maintain health under normal circumstances, but for which the body's needs will outstrip synthesis under various conditions. In the case of glutamine, fever and illness, food restriction, and other forms of physical and/or mental stress will cause the body to require more glutamine than will be available without supplementation. Under non-stressful conditions, adequate glutamine is synthesized primarily from glutamic acid, valine, and isoleucine. However, stress can drop the glutamine levels in the blood as much as 30 percent and the levels in the muscles as much as 50 percent. Glutamine is so widely used in the body that it is found in great abundance. Some authorities estimate that approximately 60 percent of the intramuscular pool of free amino acids consists of glutamine, as does 20 percent of the pool of circulating amino acids. Glutamine is the principal amino acid found in the cerebrospinal fluid.

Glutamine is used not only in the muscles but also in the metabolism of the intestinal tract, the kidneys, gallbladder, pancreas, and liver. Among amino acids, glutamine uniquely serves as a preferred energy source for rapidly dividing cells, such as those of the intestinal wall and the lymphatic system. It acts as a regulator of the body's acid-base balance—that is, it helps to maintain the proper pH of the system—through the production and removal of ammonia. This explains part of its importance for liver and brain health. When glutamic acid is combined with ammonia, it produces glutamine. Glutamine is the only amino acid that readily passes through the blood-brain barrier. It serves as a precursor to both glutamic acid, a stimulating neurotransmitter, and GABA, a calming agent. Interestingly, glutamic acid does not cross the blood-brain barrier. Glutamine is very important for muscle regeneration because it is a carrier of nitrogen between tissues and because it is an important precursor to nucleic acids, nucleotides, amino sugars, and proteins.

Physical stress, mental stress, and illness all deplete the body's glutamine stores. Authorities typically suggest supplementing with 2–3 grams of glutamine once or twice per day. This amino acid should be taken in water on an empty stomach or in a product designed to increase uptake.

For Bodybuilders and Athletes

Glutamine is anabolic, regenerative, and induces the release of growth hormone (GH); it aids in the synthesis of lean tissue, reduces recovery time, and encourages "cell volumization," a stimulus to muscle growth. As little as 2 grams of glutamine taken on an empty stomach can induce GH release.[113]

For Those with Digestive Tract Issues

Glutamine is the major fuel source for the cells that line the intestines. In Japan, those with ulcers may be told to take 1 gram of glutamine three times per day.[114] A teaching hospital associated with Harvard University sometimes gives adults with diarrhea 1 teaspoon of glutamine (about 4 grams) in water six times per day.

For Dieting, Depression, Anger, and Fatigue

To help control sugar cravings, glutamine can be used to provide the brain with an alternate fuel source. Depression, anger, and fatigue are common symptoms of inadequate glucose reaching the brain, but eating sugar usually makes matters worse by setting up an insulin surge. Take 1–2 teaspoons of glutamine (4–8 grams) in water in place of a sugary snack.

For Immune Health

Glutamine improves immune function and liver function.[115] Two grams once or twice a day suffices for maintenance; 4–8 grams may be taken once or twice a day during periods of stress.

Availability and Usage

The quantity of amino acids in formulas varies with the source, as does the price. The usual procedure is to gradually increase the dosage over several days until a maximal dosage has been reached. Results are obtained by taking the amino acids with adequate amounts of water on an empty stomach at bedtime, that is, two to four hours after meals. Sugars and refined carbohydrates should not be consumed in the meals eaten either before or after taking GH releasers. Most amino acids also can be taken upon arising and about one hour before meals. GABA, however, causes relaxation and should usually only be taken at night.

More is not necessarily better. Large amounts of pure amino acids will cause diarrhea, upset the stomach, and interfere with sleep. Some authorities suggest that it is best to combine 1 gram of L-arginine with 1 gram of L-ornithine at bedtime. Others suggest higher dosages, perhaps 5–6 grams. GABA is taken in dosages of only 1–2 grams. L-glycine again requires much higher dosages and should be taken according to the manufacturer's instructions. Use of GH releasers should always be cycled; the use of pure amino acids should be discontinued for at least one week per month.

As little as 2 grams of the amino acid L-glutamine may improve GH release. Between 8 and 10 grams of arginine aspartate has been shown to normalize GH release patterns in aging subjects to those of younger adults. (Fourth Annual Anti-Aging Conference, Las Vegas, 1996.)

For convenience and effectiveness, many companies now sell formulas that already combine two or more GH-releasing amino acids, usually arginine and ornithine. Other formulas contain L-carnitine (see L-CARNITINE/ACETYL-L-CARNITINE on page 19). The combination of L-arginine pyroglutamate and lysine may be more effective than L-arginine alone.

Since vitamin B_6 is necessary for the maximum effectiveness of these amino acids, it is added to some of their formulations. Other nutrients important for GH release include acetylcholine precursors, such as choline (or the more concentrated phosphatidyl choline) and vitamin B_5 (pantothenic acid), which likewise can be purchased from these companies. Recommendations for the latter are usually 3 grams of choline and 1 gram of vitamin B_5 taken in divided doses.

GABA is commonly counterfeited, so it should be purchased only from reputable firms. The alpha-ketoglutarate form of ornithine is only now becoming available, so it, too, should be purchased only after careful selection.

Research continues to uncover new GH releasers to add to the list of effective supplements. However, readers should not pursue unrealistic expectations with regard to oral GH releasers. They work best in individuals who are below the age of thirty-five and in good health. Fortunately, some, such as L-glutamine, are excellent health promoters regardless of their ultimate impact upon GH release.

Cautions

Those who are diabetic or borderline diabetic should avoid taking GH releasers, with L-glutamine being a notable exception inasmuch as it improves insulin sensitivity. Those who are in doubt should consult their physicians.

Supplemental chromium and/or vanadyl sulfate may be wise for anyone taking amino acids on a regular basis. Likewise, too much arginine/ornithine will disrupt the proper ratio of these GH releasers to the amino acid lysine in the body. This imbalance has been implicated in aggravating a preexisting herpes condition in sensitive individuals, and it may negatively affect other lysine-dependent reactions.

LIPOGENESIS INHIBITORS (INHIBITORS OF FAT PRODUCTION AND STORAGE)

Lipogenesis inhibitors are substances that slow the production of fats from the metabolism of carbohydrates and proteins. This means inhibiting, for instance, the synthesis of triglycerides and/or cholesterol, and likewise preventing the storage of fat in fat cells. Some known drugs, such as Triton, inhibit lipogenesis, but these drugs have many side effects and they lose their effectiveness with continued use. Safe and effective natural alternatives are now being discovered. One such natural alternative is (–)-hydroxycitric acid (HCA), which is usually made available combined with a mineral, as in calcium hydroxycitrate. HCA is extracted primarily from the dried pericarp (rind) of the fruit of *Garcinia cambogia,* native to South Asia. The fruits of related species of trees also produce HCA. Crude extracts of *G. cambogia* are popularly employed in cooking as flavoring and souring agents—for instance, in the preparation of curries. Garcinia extract also is used as a preservative, as a purgative for the treatment of intestinal worms and parasites, and for bilious digestive conditions.[116] Interestingly, in areas where it traditionally is used, *G. cambogia* is said to make meals more "filling." However, in the West until quite recently HCA has been a disappointment as a diet aid. Research over the past few years indicates that purity and delivery methods are at fault and that when these are corrected, HCA may at last live up to its promise.

How HCA Blocks Fat

HCA is remarkable for its ability to reduce the body's own synthesis of fats. During the normal metabolism of meals, carbohydrate calories that are neither used immediately for energy nor stored as glycogen are converted into fats in the liver by the enzyme ATP-citrate lyase. HCA inhibits this enzyme, and by doing so it also reduces the formation of acetyl-CoA, a biochemical that plays a key role in carbohydrate and fat metabolism. As a result, the production of low-density lipoprotein (LDL) and triglycerides is inhibited. The net effect is that fat production and storage is reduced. The appetite is controlled, food consumption is cut, and thermogenesis may be enhanced.[117]

HCA has been studied extensively for a period of more than two decades. Numerous animal trials conducted at major universities and described in peer-reviewed journals have demonstrated both the safety and the efficacy of HCA in inhibiting the production of fats from carbohydrate calories. The results of these trials have been so impressive that one of the world's largest pharmaceutical firms, Hoffmann-La Roche, not only sponsored much of the work, but also sought synthetic patentable versions of HCA to market as diet drugs. To date, no such synthetic products are available.

Since the desired effect is dosage-dependent, quality control is of major importance. As it turns out, it is quite difficult to establish the exact amount of HCA present in an extract. Many companies claim their products have a concentration of 50 percent HCA, while they actually have mistakenly counted tartaric, citric, and other organic acids present in the rind as part of the HCA content. Also important is the form of HCA used. In animal trials, the lactone form of HCA has proven to be less effective than the salt form. According to data from Hoffman-La Roche, the conversion rate of free HCA in solution into its lactone form is approximately 10 percent per week at low room temperature with an equilibrium point (usually 20 to 25 percent lactone) reached depending on concentration. Virtually all the pharmaceutical trials employed a pure trisodium hydroxycitrate containing no absorption-impeding gums, pectins, or other such compounds. Similarly, current thinking is that calcium as part of an HCA salt impedes absorption or otherwise reduces the activity of the compound. Readers should keep these points in mind because the forms of HCA available in the health food market seldom approach the optimal level of quality.

Current Controversies

Despite claims to the contrary, the employment of HCA for weight loss is not a modern Western pharmaceutical invention. In some parts of Malaysia, the fruit of *Garcinia* species is used to make a soup that is eaten before meals for weight loss. This is a traditional remedy in the villages, not the cities. Note that in this traditional use very large amounts of HCA are consumed via a liquid food, not small amounts via capsules. Moreover, a bowl of light soup before lunch and supper does seem to make HCA work better. HCA increases the body's own satiety signal, so it slows down the speed at which meals are eaten. This strategy gives the body a chance to respond to the signal that enough has been eaten. Never skip meals and do not take HCA in place of a meal—it requires food to work. Those who are sensitive to citric acid (for example, to oranges, tomatoes, and so on) may be sensitive to *Garcinia* extracts as well.

The best recent evidence suggests that the newly available HCA potassium salts are both much more effective for individual users and more effective for a greater percentage of users than the HCA calcium salts. Liquid *Garcinia* extracts likewise appear to be more readily absorbed and more active despite the lactone issue. Concurrent use of nutrients such as green tea extract or L-carnitine may improve results, especially when the fat content of the diet is not closely regulated. However, HCA definitely should *not* be taken at the same time as fiber (glucomman, guar gum, and so on) inasmuch as the fiber will bind the HCA.

HCA presently is very controversial as a weight-loss aid. In large part, this is because of purity and delivery issues. It also turns out that significant failings in the Hoffmann-La Roche pharmaceutical research are at fault, for these failings have led to the inappropriate use of HCA for weight loss. The proper use of HCA is explained below, but first here's the verdict on current HCA products.

All the major trials in the United States and Europe testing HCA products have yielded either marginal or negative results with regard to actual weight loss.[118] These trials have employed HCA salts from the leading suppliers of such products to the United States. In a marketing push, one company is now claiming that HCA increases brain serotonin levels based upon evidence of in vitro tests using rat brain slices.[119] The problem here is that Hoffman-La Roche long ago showed that HCA does not cross the blood-brain barrier. Even an increase in blood serum serotonin levels in vivo would be largely meaningless because peripheral serotonin is used entirely or almost entirely peripherally, that is, outside of the brain. This same company is claiming very good weight-loss results in a clinical trial using 2,800 mg of HCA per day given in three divided doses, thirty minutes before meals.[120] Unfortunately, only the protocol of the study was done in the United States. The trial was conducted entirely in India under Indian conditions with all oversight, data collection, and so on performed locally and with the participants eating a low-fat diet (25 percent or less) rather than American-style fare. Hence, this non-U.S. study and its results cannot be assumed to be valid under American conditions with American eating habits. Therefore, as of 2003, HCA as a weight-loss compound still awaits clinical validation in a trial conducted in the United States or Europe under Western conditions and Western standards of evidence.

HCA salts other than potassium, sodium, and some specialty compounds not yet on the market are mostly bound by bile acids, fiber, and/or other components in the diet and excreted from the body. Studies performed at the University of California at Berkeley with a leading potassium/calcium HCA showed that uptake on an empty stomach was only 20 percent at best under fasting conditions and that taking food thirty minutes after ingesting the HCA reduced absorption by 60 percent. Calcium appears to reduce the activity of HCA. Free HCA is extremely ionic and thus does not easily cross the intestinal wall into the bloodstream. There are several ways one might attempt to solve this issue. One way is to try to alter the ionic quality of the extract in the gut. An international patent application suggests that the inclusion of the *Garcinia* anthocyanin "garcinol" with the HCA salt makes HCA more effective, perhaps by improving uptake or by some other mechanism, although the results claimed are distinctly underwhelming.[121]

Delivering on the Promise of HCA

It is now known that Hoffman-La Roche made some major mistakes with regard to the mechanisms of action of HCA. Yes, the compound does inhibit the synthesis of fats from carbohydrates. It also does much more. HCA actually has two quite distinct actions in the body, one involving gastric emptying and satiety, the second involving the metabolism. In the case of appetite suppression, HCA slows the emptying of the stomach to make one feel fuller more quickly and longer—very important for dieters. Hoffman-La Roche maintained that all of HCA's effects upon appetite came from the activation of glucose receptors found in the liver, but data from Swiss researchers published in 2001 proves that this is not the case. The best available evidence indicates that HCA activates receptors in the stomach itself and in the duodenum, the first few inches of the small intestine. These receptors, in turn, activate cholecystokinin (CCK), which is a satiety compound produced in the body that requires the presence of food for its actions. The implication is that HCA must be fully and completely exposed to stomach receptors either just before food is ingested or with some source of carbohydrates, which activate sugar sensors. Given that the active HCA salts will bind to food components if left exposed to them, achieving significant appetite suppression is quite difficult. Without a delivery technology, the only published means of accomplishing this is to take approximately 2 grams of a potassium or potassium/calcium salt and dissolve it in about 8 ounces of tomato juice just before drinking the mixture some thirty minutes before meals. This method is inconvenient, to say the least. New technologies promise to solve this issue. (The action of HCA on gastric emptying and the delivery forms necessary to optimize the action are U.S. Patent pending.)

The metabolic effect of HCA is separable from its appetite-suppressing effect and requires several weeks to come into its own. The dosage of HCA necessary to reliably enhance energy metabolism is higher than the dosage necessary to reduce appetite and must be aimed at achieving blood levels rather than influencing stomach receptors. Human trials have demonstrated that HCA intake with a short-term reduction in caloric intake of about 15 percent led to very little weight loss, whereas a long-term (three months) intake of HCA that had no effect on appetite or caloric intake nevertheless led to slow, yet significant, weight loss. The key for most dieters is to combine these effects, effects involving both the appetite and the metabolism, into one package. Again, new delivery technologies promise to provide this solution. (Some delivery methods for improving HCA blood levels are protected under U.S. Patent 6,447,807 and others are U.S. Patent pending.)

Availability and Usage

Since all *Garcinia* products on the market are extracts and not pure HCA, consumers should look for the actual HCA content. For instance, 500 mg of calcium hydroxycitrate standardized as 50 percent HCA will provide 250 mg of actual HCA. The effective dosage of actual HCA probably begins at 1,000 mg taken two to three times per day in conjunction with a low-fat, low-alcohol, high-complex-carbohydrate diet. Three grams of HCA is a good starting dosage if derived from HCA potassium salt. There is no good evidence available to support dosages below 3 grams of HCA per day, and the authors themselves have seldom heard positive feedback with dosages below 11–12 grams of the calcium salt. HCA is included as a minor ingredient in quite a number of products as a "label palliative," but there is no reason to believe that this practice leads to any benefits. A fully reacted potassium hydroxycitrate is roughly three times as effective as is calcium hydroxycitrate. One of the authors was involved in a pilot clinical trial with morbidly obese patients weighing between roughly 200 and 400 pounds and found that 3 grams of HCA derived from 5 grams of potassium hydroxycitrate led to weight loss of about 3 pounds per week during the three weeks of the trial.

Ideally, dieters should take HCA with a small snack about an hour before lunch and supper and, if hungry, again before bedtime. This can be accomplished in several ways. The least convenient is to mix an HCA powder into 8–10 ounces of juice. Another method is to take an instant-releasing tablet or capsule with that same juice, although this requires that a sophisticated coating be applied to the HCA and that the tablet be specially formulated. Yet another method is to build a specially coated HCA into snacks, such as bars or liquids. This is not easily accomplished because HCA binds to the ingredients found in foods.

For the best results, two deliveries are required, one instant to achieve an effect in the stomach for satiety, and a second one that is controlled for release only in the small intestine to achieve maximal HCA blood levels. Purity and delivery are exceptionally important if results are to be found using HCA. *Very important: Do not take HCA with red pepper sauces or other capsaicin (capsicum)-containing supplements. Capsaicin negates the effects of HCA on gastric emptying.*

Cautions

Those who are diabetic or borderline diabetic may find that the amounts of HCA that are necessary to induce weight loss will also alter blood glucose levels. Individuals taking medication for diabetes and/or blood glucose regulation should supplement with the effective amounts and forms of HCA, especially the potassium salt, only under the supervision of a physician. This had not previously been recognized as an issue because of the poor quality of the available HCA salts and inadequate dosages. (The use of HCA for blood glucose and insulin regulation is under patent protection; U.S. Patent 6,207,714). Similarly, individuals being treated for blood pressure disorders may find that effective amounts and forms of HCA, especially the potassium salt, may augment the actions of hypotensive medications (U.S. Patent pending). Again, HCA influences the levels of circulating glucocorticoids (U.S. Patent 6,474,071, which also covers claims regarding leptin and several other hormones). Reducing the chronic levels of these compounds is usually to be desired, but individuals being treated therapeutically with cortisol, dexamethasone, or other corticosteroids may find that the effectiveness of their medications is reduced. Although HCA itself is an extremely safe compound, as the foregoing indicates, it is likely to indirectly influence the actions of several drugs.

LIPOTROPICS

The primary site of lipotropic action is the liver. By definition, lipotropics serve to prevent the accumulation of fat in that organ, and they usually aid in the detoxification of metabolic wastes and other toxins. Some lipotropics help to emulsify fats so that they can be more readily transported by the blood. Other lipotropics work more directly with the digestion process either by stimulating the liver to produce bile, which is then sent to the gallbladder, or by stimulating the gallbladder to release its stored bile into the digestive tract to help emulsify fats.

Nutrient lipotropics include the amino acid methionine, the digestive aids betaine HCl and lipase (a fat-digesting enzyme), and the substances choline and inositol. Herbal lipotropics include dandelion root, barberry, bearberry (*Arctostaphylos uva-ursa*), Oregon grape root, turmeric (curcumin), milk thistle (silymarin), wall germander (*Teucrium polium*), and many others. Several herbal lipotropics, including bearberry and turmeric, also act as insulin potentiators. Ancient Indian medical science (Ayurveda) lists guggul gum resin, an extract from the guggul plant (*Commiphora mukul*), as a weight-loss compound. Guggul is typically used in conjunction with three special herbs (*triphala* formula) to improve digestion and bowel function, or with *shilajit,* a mineral pitch noted for regulating blood sugar and liver disorders.

How Do Lipotropics Work?

As we will discuss in Chapter 5, a significant number of people who are overweight also show signs of liver malfunction. Lipotropics do not appear to have any significant impact upon lipolysis in athletes or in people of normal weight who are otherwise healthy. However, they may be of use to people with special needs. In animal experiments, for instance, dandelion root extract served to dramatically reduce weight, although this was due partly to its action as a diuretic.[122] Choline may be a "conditionally essential" nutrient in that, under conditions of high stress and/or in the absence of sufficient levels of methionine and perhaps folic acid, it is not manufactured in sufficient quantities by the body. In one study, healthy young adult men on a three-week choline-free diet showed sharp declines of tissue concentrations of choline and a 50 percent increase in a blood serum marker of liver damage.

Some individuals report a reduction of fat and cellulite from the use of lipotropics. However, the biochemical explanations for such reports, at this point, are largely theoretical. Research suggests that supplementing with choline (20 mg per kilogram of body weight) may reduce urinary carnitine losses by as much as 75 percent. Also, it should be kept in mind that carnitine works synergistically with coenzyme Q_{10} and pantethine.[123]

Other Benefits of Lipotropics[124]

- Methionine and choline help detoxify waste byproducts of protein synthesis. This may be especially important for those on high-protein diets.

- Lipotropics increase resistance to disease by stimulating the activity of the thymus gland.

- Choline, phosphatidyl choline, and other lipotropics can increase the production of lecithin in the liver, and lecithin may lower LDL and total cholesterol levels and help to prevent cholesterol deposits. Lecithin may help to raise the desirable HDL blood levels.

- Lipotropics may be useful in preventing gallstone formation.

- Inositol has been shown to help protect the nerves in diabetic neuropathy.

- Silymarin and lipoic acid protect the liver against toxins, act as antioxidants, and may improve the conversion of standard forms of vitamins—for example, the conversion of B_1 as thiamine HCl, B_2 as riboflavin, and so on, into their active coenzyme forms: B_1 as thiamine cocarboxylase, B_2 as riboflavin 5' phosphate, and so forth.

Availability and Usage

Each of the lipotropics mentioned above is available individually or in combination formulas. Effective doses for choline range from 500 to 1,500 mg in divided doses with meals. Recommended dosages for the other items are supplied by the manufacturers. The herbal lipotropics generally have even more pronounced effects than choline and inositol. (Those taking methionine must always supplement with vitamin B_6 because this vitamin is required for the proper metabolism of methionine.)

Very little evidence supports the notion that dieters will lose weight with lipotropics alone. The appropriate role for these nutrients is as a supporting actor in the weight-loss action, not as the lead. Most dieters will, however, feel better and achieve more healthful results with the inclusion of lipotropics in their diet programs.

MEAL REPLACEMENTS, DIET BEVERAGES, AND WEIGHT-LOSS TEAS

MEAL-REPLACEMENT FORMULAS

There are now many diets and diet systems that involve replacing one or two meals a day with a liquid or powdered drink mix. These 90- to 300-calorie formulas usually contain one-third of the RDA of vitamins, minerals, and various ratios of protein and carbohydrates. Keep in mind that it is not recommended to drop below 800 calories per day on any diet program, *and the lower the number of calories, the greater the need for high-quality protein.* Well-designed formulas provide the proper amount of quality protein necessary for a very-low-calorie diet. The best-selling brands at the supermarket rarely provide either enough protein or protein of high enough quality, because high-quality protein is costly. Indeed, the major ingredients of the most heavily promoted national brands often are sugars.

Meal-replacement programs are generally expensive, lack adequate fiber, and suffer from the various drawbacks discussed later in Chapter 5. Nevertheless, because individuals with long-standing weight issues commonly have lost their sense of proportion with regard to meal size, just providing one or two meals per day with strictly controlled caloric content seems to help with weight loss. However, any drastic reduction in calories will always invite rebound weight gain once the program is discontinued. Lifestyle changes are a necessity for lasting weight loss.

WEIGHT-LOSS TEAS

Herbs that act upon the liver are often the basis for weight-loss teas; such herbs are discussed under LIPOTROPICS on page 66. Teas that increase thermogenesis are discussed under THERMOGENIC AIDS on page 73. Other weight-loss teas contain herbs that produce laxative or diuretic effects upon the body. Some of the more complex formulas include herbs to curb the appetite and interfere with fat digestion. Simple diuretics should be avoided as a way to lose weight. Green tea and oolong tea are discussed under ANTIOXIDANTS on page 6.

KELP, VITAMIN B$_6$, LECITHIN, AND APPLE CIDER VINEGAR COMBINATIONS

Kelp, vitamin B$_6$, lecithin, and apple cider vinegar formulas were among the first to address weight loss at the biochemical level. Kelp contains iodine, which nourishes the thyroid gland and can raise the basal metabolic rate if the thyroid is underactive due to a lack of this mineral. Iodine is now commonly added to table salt and other food sources; therefore, this approach to weight loss is seldom needed or useful in the United States. Vitamin B$_6$ is necessary for fat metabolism, has diuretic properties, and its deficiency plays a role in some types of diabetes. Lecithin contains some lipotropic nutrients, *but only if the lecithin is of the very highest quality.* Most soy lecithin is of little use for nutritional purposes. Apple cider vinegar is reputed to have thyroid-stimulating and fat-emulsifying properties. In fact, acidic foods such as vinegar and lemon juice can strongly delay gastric emptying and reduce the after-meal blood sugar increase by as much as 30 percent.

COLLAGEN-BASED DIET LIQUIDS

Recently it has become popular to use collagen supplements, especially liquids taken before bedtime, to promote weight loss. There presently is no clinical evidence known to the authors to support this approach to dieting. Collagen is a very inexpensive and poor-quality protein that, as a major protein source on very-low-calorie diets, leads to reduced calcium, magnesium, and phosphate balances—even when compared with soy protein, itself not a balanced source of essential amino acids.[106] The short-term action of the collagen-based liquids is a substitution effect. Many or even most individuals with weight problems tend to snack before bedtime, and these snacks tend to be carbohydrates, such as breakfast cereals. Substituting any low-calorie, low-carbohydrate food likely will yield benefits similar to those of the collagen-based liquids. We suggest experimenting with a cup of a soothing and relaxing herbal tea (no sugar) combined with 500–1,000 mg of L-glutamine as an alternative. L-glutamine, unlike liquid collagen, offers substantial health benefits.

MEDIUM-CHAIN TRIGLYCERIDES (MCTS)

Medium-chain triglycerides (MCTs) have been used for many years for special purposes. MCTs are sometimes found in the nutrient mixtures of bedridden patients who are dependent upon intravenous nutrition. They were developed in part because they do not require the action of bile for digestion, but are absorbed directly through the walls of the small intestine and transported to the liver for oxidation. (As structurally altered fats, they have several carbon atoms removed from the normal structure of the long-chain triglycerides.) Although MCTs are found in nature, the MCT specialty oils are manmade.

How MCTs Burn Fat

In seriously catabolic patients, MCTs were found to help prevent the body from depleting its lean muscle tissues. Moreover, MCTs are not stored as body fat, but rather they are preferentially burned in the mitochondria of the cells to provide energy.[125] For some athletes and bodybuilders, this quality has proved useful since excess training depletes glycogen stores in the muscles, and continued training after such depletion can only take place partially through the breakdown of muscle protein for fuel. Extreme endurance athletes do not just burn fat; they burn muscle as well.

Does this mean that MCTs can help dieters? Yes, as long as there are not too many expectations. MCTs do seem to promote lipolysis (fat burning) and they appear to have a pronounced thermogenic effect.[126] Nevertheless, actual studies with clinically obese subjects have proved disappointing. The subjects lost weight, but at about the same rate as they did on other similar low-calorie diets. The thermogenic and lipolytic aspects of MCTs seem to be more significant for healthy subjects of normal weight and for those moderately overweight than for those who are clinically obese. However, MCTs do serve to protect the body's protein in the lean tissues during the use of low-calorie and low-carbohydrate diets.[127]

Availability and Usage

MCTs contain about 118 calories per tablespoon and can be added to a variety of foods in place of oils and fats. Since MCTs can cause stomach upset and diarrhea if taken in too large quantities, the dieter should begin with no more than a tablespoonful. Also, MCTs *are* still fats, even if structurally altered ones. In people with liver problems, quantities of MCTs taken on an empty stomach may raise blood lipids. Finally, like any other fat or oil, MCTs are subject to oxidation and should be taken with antioxidants.

The FDA recognizes MCTs only as nutrients. They are available in many health food stores, primarily in the sports-supplement sections. A few companies offer MCT oil and suggest its use in cooking, as a salad dressing, or from the bottle in small amounts. It is available in bottles containing 90 capsules of 1 gram each and as a liquid in a 16-fluid-ounce bottle.

PYRUVATE (PYR) AND DIHYDROXYACETONE (DHA)

Pyruvate (PYR) and dihydroxyacetone (DHA here, but not to be confused with the omega-3 fatty acid, docoshexaenoic acid, also called DHA) are linked to carbohydrate metabolism in the body. Through oxidation, they increase the body's energy reserves of ATP (adenosine triphosphate). ATP exists within cells, especially muscle cells. DHA is at the present time better known for its use in cosmetics[128] than for its use in dieting, although that may change. The oxidation of both compounds is quite complex within the body's basic energy cycle, called the Krebs cycle.

How Do PYR and DHA Work?

DHA and PYR are mentioned here because they have proven useful in some studies of very-low-calorie diets (VLCDs). These are diets consisting of between 400 and 800 calories, and usually 40–50 grams of high-quality protein. Going below 800 calories probably adds no additional weight-loss benefit. VLCDs work best if some small number of calories from carbohydrates are consumed; otherwise, the dieter's own protein tissue will be broken down to support blood glucose levels for the brain.

In one study, women followed a liquid diet of 500 calories a day, with 60 percent of the calories from carbohydrates, and less than 1 gram of fat. The subjects were given either DHA or PYR, whereas controls received a glucose polymer. After three weeks, both weight and total fat losses were greater in those taking DHA or PYR. Protein sparing was the same as in the controls. Also, there is some indication that the use of DHA and PYR in VLCDs (and afterward) may reduce the rebound gain of weight and fat stores after the diet is ended.[129] No major side effects have been discovered in the limited studies thus far conducted.

Many years ago, it was discovered that adding PYR to the diet prevented alcohol from causing animals to develop fatty livers. This suggested that the compound might have a generally positive effect on the functioning of the liver. PYR is now covered by a large number of U.S. patents that describe its use for weight loss, lowering blood fats, reducing insulin levels, increasing glycogen stores, and most recently, preventing free-radical generation (U.S. Patents 4,812,479; 4,874,790; 5,134,162; and 5,480,909). In animal studies, PYR has been shown to increase both thermogenesis and general energy expenditure. Even the rate of synthesis of new fat in fat cells appears to be affected by PYR, although the reasons for this are unclear.

The major drawback with the use of PYR in weight loss is the large amount required. The dosage listed in the patents runs from 2 to 15 percent of the total calories in the diet, and this presumes the concurrent ingestion of a low-fat diet. Translated into human dietary terms, this means the intake for proven efficacy with PYR begins at about 20 grams per day, under the best of conditions, and ranges up to more than 50 grams. Whether this threshold can be lowered and the proven benefits of PYR increased through other means is still being explored. It has been suggested that dosages in the range of 6 grams may prove effective. However, this 6-gram dosage is based upon extrapolations from changes in animal response curves and not upon human data. Obviously, no dieter can take 20–50 grams of PYR per day. And, indeed, PYR has failed in the market at the lower dosage.

Availability and Usage

The version of PYR in which the compound is stabilized with calcium is preferable to the one stabilized with sodium, so purchasers should read the fine print and look for the ingredient "calcium pyruvate." Instructions for use will be found on the products, but at this point it appears that the original dosage recommendations of 20–50 grams per day are justified. This high level of intake tended to cause gastrointestinal distress in subjects in the clinical trials and is far beyond what most dieters can either afford or routinely supplement. As for DHA, this has not appeared in commercial formulations.

THERMOGENIC AIDS

Thermogenesis is an increase in the body's production of heat energy, triggered by nutritional and biochemical means. One of the chief drawbacks of calorie-restricted diets is their tendency to lower the body's rate of energy production. Thermogenic aids can help correct this. Common aids include caffeine, L-phenylalanine, L-tyrosine, the Chinese herb ma huang, L-carnitine, yohimbe, and other products.

How Thermogenic Compounds Help with Weight Loss

As we will discuss in Chapter 5, individuals prone to obesity often have lower basal metabolic rates (BMRs), and obesity itself promotes a lowering of the BMR. After eating, most people see a lasting rise in energy production amounting to 10 to 20 percent of their prior metabolic rates. For reasons not well understood, overweight women in particular do not experience this increase in heat production.[130]

Certain naturally occurring substances, such as ephedrine contained in the herb ma huang, speed up the resting metabolic rate, act as stimulants, and suppress the appetite. Caffeine and other members of the xanthine family have similar effects and can be found in coffee, kola nut, tea, yerba maté, and many other herbal teas and foods. The seaweed known as bladderwrack (*Fucus*) activates the thyroid and has been used in Europe to treat obesity and hypothyroidism since the seventeenth century. Bladderwrack may be less useful in the modern period, now that table salt is routinely enriched with iodine.

Many of the substances listed in the section on appetite suppressants also act to raise the metabolic rate. L-phenylalanine and L-tyrosine perform this function by serving as precursors to epinephrine and norepinephrine, that is, as precursors to adrenaline and noradrenaline. High-protein diets, which supply these amino acids, will tend to speed up bodily processes in general. Since thyroid activators often produce results similar to adrenal stimulants, the following section, THYROID NUTRIENTS AND ACTIVATORS on page 80, is also important. Thyroid hormone and norepinephrine both activate the heat-producing tissue called brown fat, or brown adipose tissue. Also of great importance is the need to prevent the suppression of the action of the lipolytic and brown-fat-activating hormone *glucagon* by insulin (released by the consumption of carbohydrates). Brown fat is discussed in greater detail in Chapter 5.

It should be noted that caffeine, ephedrine, and related products should not be consumed in excess. They make susceptible individuals nervous and activate a feedback circuit involving the thyroid.

New studies have revealed yet another thermogenic herb, or rather a new use for an old substance. It seems that yohimbine hydrochloride, an extract from the bark of the yohimbe tree, not only is, at least partially, the male sexual stimulant tradition claims that it is, but also is able to increase the release of noradrenaline. This action "stimulates the system, raises body temperature, and causes the body to mobilize fat for fuel. Yohimbine appears to be effective in all these areas."[131] In one study, patients given 15 mg of yohimbine hydrochloride per day on a 1,000-calorie-a-day diet lost an average of 7.8 pounds in three weeks, in comparison with 4.8 pounds lost by the control subjects.[132] There are other thermogenic aids in the plant kingdom as well, such as mustard seed and cayenne pepper. These last two items help to begin the thermogenic process and make other substances, including caffeine and ephedrine, more effective as thermogenic aids.

Caffeine and ephedrine work better taken together than either one taken alone. Ephedrine mimics many of the effects of the release of adrenaline from the adrenal glands. Caffeine, which stimulates the pituitary directly and the thyroid indirectly, stimulates the adrenals through the action of the thyroid. The theophylline found in tea also opens up the peripheral capillaries to a certain extent. This means that the heat generated by thermogenesis can be dissipated. Fat acts as an insulator and thereby usually causes the body to turn off heat production. Some diet formulas add additional antipyretics such as aspirin or white willow bark in order to further dissipate the heat produced by thermogenic stimulants. Antipyretics are essential for safe thermogenesis. Antioxidants, likewise, are necessary for the safe long-term use of thermogenic products inasmuch as such stimulation increases free-radical production. Interestingly, the antioxidant polyphenols found in tea, such as the catechins, and not just the caffeine and theophylline, also may improve thermogenesis. It has been known for thirty years that catechins slow the destruction of the body's adrenaline. Now it has been shown in tissue studies that tea extracts without caffeine can stimulate thermogenesis in brown fat and that the effect is stronger when ephedrine is added.[133] Other compounds, such as the flavonoid naringen, are sometimes added to formulas to delay the destruction of adrenaline and noradrenaline or to prevent the downregulation of cAMP (cyclic adenosine monophosphate)-controlled energy regulation within the cells, and therefore increase the response to ephedrine.

A quite common formulation of thermogenic herbs is as an ECA "stack," where ECA stands for ephedrine, caffeine, and aspirin. All three of these ingredients can come from a variety of different natural sources as well as from synthetic products. Although ma huang is the chief natural source of the ephedrine family of compounds, there are other minor sources, such as *Sida cordifolia*. Sadly, herbal extracts supplying ephedrine alkaloids are fairly commonly "spiked" with synthetic pseudoephedrine.[134] More positively, ma huang contains one or more still unidentified compounds that extend the active life of ephedrine through a mechanism similar to that of caffeine.[135] Only a full-spectrum extract, usually standardized for no more than 6 percent ephedrine alkaloids, will contain all of these compounds.

The primary benefit of ephedrine-based combinations is a reduction in appetite rather than thermogenesis. For most individuals, between 75 and 80 percent of the impact of taking an ephedrine and caffeine product will come from appetite suppression for at least the first four weeks of use, and perhaps as long as the first eight weeks of use. Furthermore, it should be pointed out that no clinical trial has ever been undertaken to prove that ephedrine plus caffeine plus aspirin gives results superior to ephedrine plus caffeine, nor has it been shown conclusively that aspirin is superior to a properly calibrated amount of willow bark extract in these formulas.

At fairly high dosages, versions of the ECA stack can cause a significant increase in the number of calories burned per day. In one test, 50 mg of ephedrine was given to volunteers three times per day. Under controlled conditions and using very precise monitors to measure energy expenditure, it was found that 3.6 percent more energy was expended in a twenty-four-hour period when the subjects were taking the ephedrine.[136] A similar experiment conducted using 22 mg of ephedrine plus 30 mg caffeine and 50 mg theophylline three times per day provided better results than those found with ephedrine alone. This combination increased the number of calories burned by 8 percent per day.[137] These results give an indication of the impact of caffeine in extending the life of ephedrine in the body.

Because there are many potential side effects linked to the use of ephedra alkaloids, many have attempted to find a suitable substitute for ephedrine. Widely used at this point are extracts of the dried immature fruit of bitter orange (*Citrus aurantium,* Chinese zhi shi); one proprietary extract claims to include all five active compounds found in this fruit, synephrine being perhaps the most important of these compounds. One study combined 975 mg of *Citrus aurantium* extract with 528 mg of caffeine and 900 mg of St. John's wort (a catechin source) for use with an 1,800-kilocalorie-a-day diet. At the end of six weeks, the subjects taking the active ingredients had lost 1.5 percent of their starting body weight (about 3.1 pounds), a result that was statistically significant. These findings suggest that synephrine, when taken together with the other compounds found in *Citrus aurantium,* is useful in weight loss.[138] As we will see shortly, a more appropriate combination of supplements likely would have doubled these results.

Citrus aurantium has been shown in animal studies to increase the metabolism of fat while improving physical performance and helping to protect lean tissue. Compared with ephedrine, *Citrus aurantium* extract shows less effect upon appetite and more effect upon thermogenesis while exhibiting very little impact upon the central nervous or cardiovascular systems. In fact, *Citrus aurantium* in at least one model actually reduced portal vein pressure, a symptom of a particular type of high blood pressure.[139] *Citrus aurantium* extract stimulates the thermogenic beta-3 adrenergic receptors, yet has little effect upon the alpha-1 and alpha-2 receptors or upon the beta-1 and beta-2 receptors. Both latter sets of receptors are responsible for the pressor effect (blood-pressure-raising effect) and the central nervous system side effects found with ephedrine. Unlike the ephedrine alkaloids found in ma huang, the active amines of *Citrus aurantium* extract do not readily cross the blood-brain barrier.

The actions of the adrenal stimulants—regardless of the source—can be increased indirectly through supplements that contain the building blocks for adrenal hormones, for example L-tyrosine. This approach has the advantage of helping to prevent thyroid and adrenal exhaustion. Exhaustion of the sympathetic nervous system can be avoided through the addition of hawthorn berry, licorice, and magnesium to formulas. The health of the adrenal glands and the parasympathetic nervous system can be safeguarded by the addition of acetylcholine precursors such as DMAE (dimethylaminoethanol) and vitamin B_5 (pantothenic acid or its coenzyme, pantethine).

Spicy Foods for a Metabolic Boost

If you want to boost your metabolism, but would rather not take pills that may increase your blood pressure, there is a way. Adding a bit of spice to meals can accomplish more than just giving zest to bland foods. Spices can both increase total calories burned and help us to metabolize fat for energy. Fat, of course, is the stuff we tend to add to our midsections. If we eat fat, our options are to either burn it or wear it. Recent studies have shown that dietary red pepper, such as the fiery liquid that comes in little bottles, can significantly boost diet-induced thermogenesis and increase the oxidation of fat for energy. Similar effects can be achieved with a constituent found in mustard. The pungent principles in ginger also increase metabolism, but by different mechanisms. An added bonus is that all three of these spices improve digestion. A report in the press in 1999 described a study done at Oxford Polytechnic Institute in England in which dieters who added 1 teaspoon each of hot-pepper sauce and mustard to every meal raised their metabolic rate by as much as 25 percent. Those who want to try the spicy-diet approach might take 1 teaspoon of red-pepper hot sauce and 1 teaspoon of spicy prepared mustard in the middle of each meal.[140] (The hot Chinese mustard is too strong for most people at this level of intake.) If the meal does not include ginger, follow the meal with a cup of ginger tea. However, if eating late in the evening, do not add this much spice; raising your metabolism very late in the day will interfere with sleep.

Availability and Usage

Thermogenic aids have become quite common as diet aids. They work so successfully that pharmaceutical research is now being directed toward this weight-loss approach. A new class of drugs called thermogenic beta-3 agonists is being developed in Europe to perform as thermogenic aids. However, these are not expected to be available until the end of this decade.[141]

Realistically, substitutes for ephedrine do not work nearly as well as ephedrine itself. This is due to the fact that most of the weight lost with ephedrine products is through appetite suppression. Bitter orange extracts, for instance, although boasting much or all of the thermogenic impact of ephedrine, lack the appetite-controlling aspect of that compound.

Yohimbe products are widely available, but most are lacking in the active ingredient. As with all herbs, only buy products with guaranteed potencies or other forms of standardization.

Cautions

No strong stimulants should be used by individuals with conditions including (but not limited to) high blood pressure, diabetes, heart disease, kidney disease, liver disease, neurological disease, and epilepsy. Women with fibrocystic breast disease should avoid xanthines as they may aggravate this condition. Caution should be exercised in mixing sources of caffeine and ephedrine, or these two with L-phenylalanine, L-tyrosine, or yohimbe. Taken together in excess, these combinations can lead to nervousness, excitability, insomnia, and nausea. Moreover, long-term usage of large amounts of adrenal mimics and stimulants may be undesirable, especially in the absence of nutrients that support the health of the adrenal gland and the nervous system (see THYROID NUTRIENTS AND ACTIVATORS on page 80). Traditional systems of herbal treatment commonly add herbs such as licorice and hawthorn to strong stimulant formulas in order to reduce negative side effects. Thermogenesis inducers should be cycled five to six days on and one to two days off per week and also three weeks on and one week off per month. Yohimbe poses a number of special problems in that it may be undesirable for use by individuals with various psychosomatic disorders, thyroid issues, blood pressure problems, or gastrointestinal-tract ulcers or disorders.

The potential for the development of psychological dependence and abuse of ephedrine products is very high. Individuals should carefully monitor how they interact with these and other strong stimulants. In some areas, such as in bodybuilding and among adolescents, abuse is extremely common.[142]

And a Further Warning

In September 1992, the FDA issued an import bulletin on the herb ephedra, an opening round of the FDA's effort to reclassify ephedra as an "unapproved food additive," or otherwise restrict its use. Since that time, the FDA has revoked the over-the-counter (OTC) status of at least one related compound, phenylpropanolamine (PPA), which once was sold freely for weight loss. At the time of this writing, eight states have banned the sale of ephedrine in herbal and other forms, except by way of prescription, and more states are expected to follow suit. In early 2003, the FDA proposed that the following primary warning should be mandated for all products containing ephedrine alkaloids:

> **Contains ephedrine alkaloids.** Heart attack, stroke seizure, and death have been reported after consumption of ephedrine alkaloids. Not for pregnant or breast-feeding women or persons under age eighteen. Risk or injury can increase with dose or if used during strenuous exercise or with other products containing stimulants (including caffeine). Do not use with certain medications or if you have certain health conditions. Stop use and contact a doctor if side effects occur.

On December 30, 2003, the FDA formally indicated that it intended to seek a complete ban on the free sale of ephedra-containing products.

Questions of safety continue to be debated. A recently released study found that ephedrine plus caffeine in a six-month trial was safe in otherwise healthy overweight subjects (subjects' total daily dose of ephedra was 90 mg; daily dose of caffeine was 192 mg).[143] To put the safety issue in perspective, according to one estimate, everyday foods are linked to approximately 5,000 deaths per year, prescription and other drugs most recently to 1,418 deaths per year, and the entire dietary supplements industry to about twelve deaths per year (*Whole Foods* magazine, October 2003). Ephedrine products have been and continue to be very widely used in weight-loss formulas and, to be sure, also account for the majority of complaints associated with the ingestion of dietary supplements. Nevertheless, the safety concerns presented to the public by the FDA with regard to ephedrine appear to go well beyond the data currently available.

THYROID NUTRIENTS AND ACTIVATORS: GUGGUL, FORSKOLIN, AND PHOSPHATES

The thyroid is an endocrine gland located in the neck. It produces two hormones, thyroxine (also called tetraiodothyronine, or T4) and triiodothyronine (T3), which are responsible for various functions in the body. These hormones increase protein synthesis in all body tissues, and they increase the activity of NA/K ATPase enzymes. These latter enzymes influence the rate at which fat is burned for energy. If the thyroid is not functioning properly, a slow metabolism can result. Thus, many people with underactive thyroids also have weight problems. And thyroid dysfunction is often involved in menstrual difficulties.

A common method for testing thyroid function is to place a thermometer under the arm for ten minutes before getting out of bed in the morning. The thermometer must read to tenths of a degree. Normal body temperature ranges for this test are between 97.8 and 98.2 degrees Fahrenheit. Readings below 97.8°F may indicate hypothyroid (low thyroid) activity, and readings above 98.2°F may indicate hyperthyroid (excess thyroid) activity.

Some of the factors that can cause thyroid problems (thereby decreasing the rate at which the body burns calories) include malnourishment of the thyroid through vitamin and mineral deficiencies; thyroid and/or pituitary exhaustion as a result of overstimulation with caffeine, sugar, and other stimulants; and the presence of substances that inhibit thyroid function, such as alcohol.

The Thyroid's Role in Obesity

Most people associate the thyroid gland with iodine, and iodine is important. However, thyroid functioning benefits from good nutrition in general. Deficiencies of vitamins A, B_2, C, and E have all been linked to thyroid insufficiency. Moreover, there is a link between thyroid malfunction and the inability either to absorb some nutrients (for example, vitamin B_{12}) or to transform others into their active forms (for example, the transformation of beta-carotene into vitamin A).[144] Since the use of supplemental thyroid hormones requires the supervision of a doctor, this is a case in which an ounce of prevention is worth a pound of cure.

The thyroid's regulatory function is commonly damaged through the excessive consumption of caffeine, sugar and, other simple carbohydrates. These act as pituitary stimulants, and the pituitary, in turn, stimulates the release of thyroid hormones. Excessive stimulation of the pituitary ultimately damages that gland's ability to produce the hormone necessary to activate the thyroid, whereas serotonin, the hormone that reduces thyroid activity, continues to be produced.

Whatever the source of hypothyroidism, the effects are the same. Inadequate thyroid hormone secretion causes the adrenal glands to fail to secrete enough cortisol. Without adrenal cortisol, the liver does not produce and store enough glycogen, an essential storage sugar that the liver releases in a controlled manner to maintain balanced blood sugar levels. As a result, hypothyroidism can lead to a feeling of sluggishness and lassitude as well as cravings for sugars and other simple carbohydrates.[145]

A good thyroid-support formula should combine L-tyrosine (a precursor to the thyroid hormones) with the following: magnesium, potassium, zinc, manganese, iodine, vitamin B_1 (thiamine), vitamin B_2 (riboflavin), vitamin B_3 (niacin), vitamin B_6, and the antioxidant vitamins A, C, and E. The seaweed known as bladderwrack is one of several herbs noted for specific thyroid support, albeit this may be largely due to its iodine content. Most of these vitamins and minerals help transform L-tyrosine into thyroid and adrenal hormones. Low thyroid function is often reflective of poor general nutrition.

Dieters should also read the earlier discussion on gamma-linolenic acid (GLA) and the omega-3 fatty acids. These "good" fats improve thyroid function and are essential for thermogenesis. (See GAMMA-LINOLENIC ACID (GLA), FLAX, AND THE OMEGA-3 ESSENTIAL FATTY ACIDS on page 48.)

Thyroid Activators—What Are They and How Do They Work?

There are relatively few safe direct activators of the thyroid. Two herbal compounds with some good scientific evidence behind claims of their effectiveness are guggul and *Coleus forskohlii* extract. Phosphate salts may prevent the reduction in thyroid hormone activity normally caused by reduced-calorie diets.

Guggul

The special Ayurvedic compound known as guggul (a gum resin derived from the guggul tree, *Commiphora mukul*), standardized as guggulipid

(25 mg guggulsterones per gram) has been shown to have a dramatic impact upon cholesterol and triglyceride levels, as well as being an aid to weight loss. Clinical studies have found that total cholesterol, LDL (low-density lipoprotein) and VLDL (very-low-density lipoprotein) cholesterol, and triglycerides all can be reduced by approximately 30 percent through the use of a standardized source of guggul (guggulipid), yet the fraction of desirable HDL (high-density lipoprotein) cholesterol actually increases as much as 36 percent as a result of using this gum resin. When the smaller amount of guggulipid that is necessary for weight loss was used in a trial, there were 7 to 11 percent reductions for the bad blood fats and a 5 to 6 percent elevation of the good HDL. When using Ayurvedic weight-loss formulas for a period of three months, non-dieting subjects lost 12.1–12.7 pounds more than those taking a placebo.[146] Trials using guggulipid alone without any other herbs indicated that as little as 200 mg taken three times per day before meals caused weight loss in overweight subjects. The effective dosage may vary if combined with other ingredients, such as *shilajit* (see LIPOTROPICS on page 66). These results were achieved under non-American conditions. In the United States, guggul extracts appear to be more successful as components of more extensive formulas.

Guggul with Phosphates

A good combination is guggul with various phosphate salts. The thyroid-activating and weight-loss stimulation of this combination is covered by patent (U.S. Patent 6,113,949). The principal ingredients in this product are guggulsterone, phosphate salts, and the amino acid L-tyrosine (a building block for thyroid hormone and certain neurotransmitters). In European trials, phosphate supplementation has been proven to prevent the reduction in thyroid action and energy metabolism that usually is found with dieting. In a clinical trial, this patented product led to weight loss of just under a pound per week.

Phosphates

Phosphate salts appear to prevent the reduction in the conversion of T4 to T3 that is normally caused by very-low-calorie diets. T3 is the metabolically and energetically more active of the two major thyroid hormones. Hence, a reduction in T3 levels due to a reduced intake of calories also leads to a reduction in expended energy and a general slowing down of the metabolism. Many researchers consider T3 to be a key to weight-loss plateaus and to the body's "set point" for weight and energy expenditure. In one study, thirty overweight women participated in an eight-week slimming program consisting of a self-controlled, low-energy diet supplemented with highly viscous fibers and mineral tablets containing calcium, potassium, and sodium phosphates. Although there were no great differences in weight loss caused by these salts, during periods of phosphate supplementation, the resting metabolic rate (RMR) increased by approximately 12 percent in one group and 19 percent in a second group. Both results were statistically significant. Phosphate supplementation ameliorated a decrease in plasma T3 level and a decrease in T4 to T3 ratio.[147] No one holds that supplementation with phosphates alone induces a great deal of weight loss, yet it is significant to find that phosphates can prevent the thyroid downregulation typical of diets. Approximately 3 grams of mixed phosphate salts appears to be required for this effect.

Forskolin

The active components of *Coleus forskohlii* (chiefly forskolin) are pharmacologically quite significant in their effects. One of forskolin's modes of action is to activate adenylate cyclase, which in turn increases the amount of cyclic adenosine monophosphate (cAMP) operating in cells. Quite simply, this improves the capacity of cells to respond to signals carried by thyroid and adrenal hormones. Perhaps the best-researched aspect of forskolin is its ability to encourage lipolysis, the release of fatty acids from storage. Not only does forskolin activate adipocyte (fat cell) lipolysis, but it also reduces the synthesis of fat in adipocytes. This may be in part due to its effect of inhibiting the transport of glucose into fat cells. Alternatively, it may be the case that forskolin acts through a synergism with lipolytic (fat-releasing) hormones. Again, increased levels of cAMP may improve the impact of thyroid hormones on the uncoupling protein found in brown adipose tissue, and hence improve thermogenesis. The result of supplementation with forskolin is a tendency to increase the ratio of lean to fat tissue in the body. Other possible benefits include improved mood and immune response.

As is often the case, there are plant speciation issues with members of the *Coleus* family. Moreover, there are extraction issues. Therefore, few reliable sources of forskolin are available. One such source is Sabinsa

Corporation, the patent holder for the extract sold as ForsLean (U.S. Patent 5,804,596). The patent describes the use of a standardized 10 percent forskolin extract for increasing lean body mass. In this case, the supplier, as the patent holder, has a vested interest in the product's working as claimed.[148] Those who are connected to the Internet can explore the science behind ForsLean at http://www.forslean.com/home.htm. The typical dosage is 250 mg (yielding 25 mg forskolin) taken twice a day.

CHAPTER 3

The Anti-Fat Nutrient Weight-Loss Program

O UR CORE PROGRAM FOCUSES ON THREE COMPONENTS: essential fatty acids, fiber, and protein. In a nutshell, this means supplementing with the "good" fats, adding fiber to the diet (preferably in the form of lightly cooked green vegetables), and increasing the percentage of calories derived from good-quality protein sources. These are the primary players on the weight-loss stage. Other supplements—the most important being L-glutamine, acetyl-L-carnitine, and alpha-lipoic acid— play supporting roles. The reason for this is that we are recommending permanent lifestyle changes that dieters can follow not just to lose weight, but to avoid continuously regaining excess pounds. Moreover, the Anti-Fat Nutrient Weight-Loss Program is a "food-based" approach, which easily can be turned into a more insulin-sensitizing and thermogenic program through the simple addition of herbs and spices.

"Good" fats are the first component of the program. (To refresh your memory, you may wish to reread GAMMA-LINOLENIC ACID (GLA), FLAX, AND THE OMEGA-3 ESSENTIAL FATTY ACIDS on page 48 in Chapter 2.) For a large percentage of those who are over their ideal weights, essential fatty acids, taken together, constitute the most important single supplement— they are really a food more than a supplement. In obesity, the body's synthesis of the omega-6 fatty acid gamma-linolenic acid (GLA) tends to be below par, and the intake of omega-3 fatty acids from flaxseed and fish is almost always inadequate. GLA affects the production of a whole series of hormones, and through these it plays a significant role in fat metabolism. Many of our modern processing techniques for oils and other foods seriously interfere with the body's production and utilization of GLA, just as omega-3 fatty acids are poorly represented in modern diets. Dieters should strive to achieve a 2:1 ratio in their intake of omega-6 to omega-3 fatty acids. After sufficient weight loss, the ratio may be increased to 3:1.

Although it is possible to overconsume omega-3 fatty acids, to do so is very rare via Western diets. Omega-3 fats tend to be largely absent from the modern food supply and therefore may require supplementation.

Fiber is the second component of the program. (Again, you may wish to reread FIBER on page 46 in Chapter 2.) For literally decades, researchers have remarked that the ratio of carbohydrate to fat to protein in the diet seemed to be much less important in determining body weight than the caloric density of the diet. Fat happens to be calorically dense; however, in the Mediterranean region of Europe the traditional diets derive 40 percent of their calories from fats, yet this has never been associated with weight gain. The reason is that these diets are characterized by the consumption of soups, multiple small courses, and lots of vegetables, which are included to provide taste, color, and texture to Mediterranean cuisine. Worldwide, there just is no consistent association between the amount of fat in the diet and weight gain. Although a great deal of support has long been available for the idea that meal volume and, as a related factor, the speed of meal consumption both play crucial roles in satiety, validation has come in great detail through the work of Barbara Rolls at Penn State University. Through a large number of experiments, Dr. Rolls has proven that very simple means can be used to reduce daily caloric intake while actually increasing meal satisfaction. At its simplest, this means consuming a bowl of light soup before lunch and supper and including high-volume foods, primarily vegetables, as the major component of meals. Tasty, healthful, and painless! Unfortunately, only between 10 and 20 percent of Americans consume the mere five servings of fruits and vegetables each day that is recommended by health authorities. Those interested in reading about the food-volume approach in depth should consult *The Volumetrics Weight-Control Plan* by Barbara Rolls, Ph.D., and Robert A. Barnett (HarperCollins, 2000).

Protein is the third component of the triad underlying our weight-loss approach. As a matter of historical record, protein intake in the United States has remained fairly consistent at between 12 and 15 percent of calories for as far back as we have good records, that is to say, for roughly 150 to 200 years. Massive weight gain throughout the general populace has occurred only in the last forty years, hence a change in protein intake by itself is not an answer to why Americans are now so overweight. Nevertheless, various studies have consistently shown that caloric restriction is much easier on diets in which protein accounts for 25 to 35 percent of calories. In the suggested starting diet given in this chapter, the authors present an approach in which breakfast and one other meal each day are very heavily weighted toward an increased intake of protein. Protein tends to improve thyroid function and to increase thermogenesis, so there are many advantages to the dieter. Some subcomponents of protein sources, such as L-glutamine, improve the release of growth hormone and help to prevent weight gain on poorly designed high-fat diets.

Beyond these general suggestions, it must be pointed out that individuals gain weight for different reasons having to do with their metabolic individuality and the lives they lead. For instance, those who eat to control nervousness may be helped more by herbal anxiolytics than by any full-scale frontal attack upon their waistlines (see the antistress nutrients to follow in this chapter). Thermogenesis-inducing items, such as caffeine and ephedrine, may not be useful for those who are already prone to nervousness or for those who exhibit pituitary-related hypothyroidism; yet for those suffering from simple cases of dieting-induced sluggish metabolisms, such items may prove effective. (The authors much prefer the use of thermogenic spices to the use of strong stimulants.)

It is suggested that every dieter take a good vitamin and mineral supplement to provide nutritional insurance. The antioxidant vitamins and plant antioxidants should be well represented through other specialty supplements. Some plant sources of antioxidants, such as green tea and oolong tea or even extracts from grape seeds, help to increase the daily expenditure of calories and therefore might be emphasized for additional benefits.

Mineral supplementation should emphasize chromium, copper, magnesium, manganese, potassium, and zinc. These are especially important to dieters, but they are more broadly useful in controlling blood pressure and insulin response. Magnesium, zinc, and the vitamins B_3, B_6, and C are necessary for the conversion of polyunsaturated fats in the diet into hormones. Magnesium and potassium are necessary for the activation of brown adipose tissue (brown fat) for thermogenesis.

Two nutrients should be given a second look for other reasons. Vitamin B_6, which is easily destroyed in cooking of any sort, is important for protein metabolism and synthesis, and it has been shown to have an impact on some forms of diabetes.[1] Moreover, it also has been demonstrated that men (more so than women) in their sixties can rapidly be made much less insulin sensitive (that is, nonreactive to insulin) by being fed a diet lacking in vitamin B_6.[2] A chromium deficiency is linked even more strongly to blood sugar problems than is a deficiency in vitamin B_6. This mineral directly affects the body's response to insulin.

Indeed, one of the classic dysfunctions that appears with age and also with obesity is the reversal of the quantities of two antagonistic hormones produced by the body: insulin and growth hormone (GH). On the one hand, insulin (which stores calories as fats and controls blood sugar levels) is produced in only small amounts when we are young, and we do not need much at that time since in youth our tissues are quite sensitive to insulin. On the other hand, GH is abundantly produced in the bodies of teenagers and young adults, and this is one of the reasons that is used to be young people could "eat anything" and still not get fat. The experience of the last decade shows that even this advantage can be undermined by the modern American diet and lack of exercise.

Unfortunately, GH release gradually declines after the age of thirty. Excess fat storage itself upsets the body's hormonal balance and depresses the production of GH. As we age we also tend to produce more insulin because our tissues become less sensitive to its effects. One side effect of excessive insulin production and insulin tolerance is the tendency to put on weight. By adding the vitamins B_6 and C, and the mineral chromium to the diet, we can better affect both the production of GH and the regulation of insulin.

RESULTS IN FIFTEEN DAYS

Any well-designed nutrient-based diet program should be given two to three weeks to produce results. For instance, a well-designed thermogenic product that incorporates the herbs and supporting nutrients described in the previous chapter will work better the second week than during the first, and better the third week than during the second. The reason for this is that your body has a great deal of built-in inertia or resistance to change. However, with the proper approach almost any dieter can expect to take off and keep off 1 to 2 pounds per week during the first three to four weeks while actually improving energy levels and muscle tone. Give your chosen program at least two weeks to begin to deliver results, and judge yourself by how you feel and how you look rather than by numbers on the bathroom scale alone.

FAT-BURNING PRODUCTS

Numerous vitamin and pharmaceutical companies now are selling weight-control products based on the anti-fat nutrients described in this book. These formulas are getting better all the time and there are some quite effective fat-burning products on the market. These products usually consist of multi-nutrient tablets that include some of the anti-fat nutrients. Due to size limitations, it is difficult to include effective amounts of more than one anti-fat nutrient category in such a tablet. For example, some products contain mostly lipotropics, whereas others provide primarily thermogenic nutrients. While you can obtain a measure of success by using just one special nutrient or category of nutrients, results can be enhanced by using a variety of anti-fat nutrients at the same time. Whether you choose to use one of these products, design your own program, or use the program that follows, you should make yourself familiar with the nutrients in Chapter 2.

The following program is based on the experiences of the authors as nutritional consultants. A physician should be consulted before starting any nutrition or exercise program. Before taking any of the following nutrients, please read Chapter 2 for important additional information. Also see Chapter 2 for potencies of nutrients in instances where they are not mentioned here.

THE CORE PROGRAM

In the next chapter we'll discuss the five principles of weight loss and the three keys of optimal "food coupling," which will allow you to plan nutritious meals that will give you energy without adding pounds. With the information provided, you will have plenty of freedom to choose the foods you eat without severe limitations. Here we are presenting the heart of our nutrient-based fat-loss plan, which you will integrate with "properly coupled" meals of your own choosing:

Thirty Minutes Before Breakfast

- 1 glass of water (not chilled) with 1 tablespoon of crushed or ground flaxseeds;

- 2,000 milligrams (mg) of L-glutamine (bulk powder can be added to the drink);

- 1,000 mg of acetyl-L-carnitine (capsule); and

- 300 mg of alpha-lipoic acid (sustained release).

With Breakfast

- A multivitamin and mineral supplement;
- 200 micrograms (mcg) of chromium;
- 240 mg of GLA;
- 1,000 mg of omega-3 EPA/DHA (80 percent concentration from fish oils); and
- Thermogenic spices.

Mid Morning

- 1 glass of water (not chilled) with 2 teaspoons of spirulina or green barley grass extract; and
- 1,000 mg of acetyl-L-carnitine (capsule).

With Lunch

- A multivitamin and mineral supplement; and
- Thermogenic spices.

Mid Afternoon

- 1 glass of water (not chilled) with 2 teaspoons of spirulina or green barley grass extract; and
- Whole fruit (for example, an apple or orange) or vegetable snack (for example, carrot, celery, or zucchini sticks).

Thirty Minutes Before Dinner

- 1 glass of water (not chilled) with 1 tablespoon crushed or ground flaxseeds; and
- 2,000 mg of L-glutamine (bulk powder can be added to the drink).

With Dinner

- A multivitamin and mineral supplement;
- 200 mcg of chromium;
- 240 mg of GLA;
- 1,000 mg of omega-3 EPA/DHA (80 percent concentration from fish oils); and
- Thermogenic spices (omit if these interfere with sleep).

Late Evening

Avoid carbohydrate snacks within three hours of bedtime; limit or avoid alcohol during this same period. Dieters who routinely are hungry before bedtime are not consuming enough calories during the day. In place of a bowl of cereal, try a cup of chamomile tea supplemented with 1–2 grams of L-glutamine. Another acceptable snack is 1 tablespoon of flax (ground or cracked) or psyllium husk powder in a large glass of unchilled water (this suggestion comes from Ann Louise Gittleman's *The Fat Flush Plan*).

AUGMENTING WEIGHT-LOSS NUTRIENTS

In Chapter 5 we will see that false hunger can occur from low blood sugar, from stress and anxiety, from depression and boredom, and from nutrient deficiencies, which can all come from eating refined foods (including white sugar, white flour products, and white rice). The following nutrients can help each of these conditions.

Anti-Sugar-Craving Nutrients

Adequate dietary protein, complex carbohydrates, chromium (minimum dose 400 mcg per day in divided doses); alpha-lipoic acid (100–600 mg per day); L-glutamine (1–2 grams, three times per day between meals).

Antistress/Anxiolytic Nutrients

Magnesium, B vitamins, vitamin C, DMAE, pantothenic acid, L-theanine (100–200 mg per day), valerian herb extract, passion flower extract, chamomile tea, chrysin (500 mg).

Anti-Depression Nutrients

L-phenylalanine, L-tyrosine, *Ginkgo biloba* herb, L-glutamine (1–2 grams, three times per day between meals), 5-HTP, SAMe.

Anti-Appetite Nutrients

Fiber, 5-HTP, L-phenylalanine, L-tyrosine, thermogenic supplements, extra water, L-glutamine (1–2 grams, three times per day between meals).

Partitioning Nutrients

Forskolin extract (equivalent to 25 mg forskolin twice per day), CLA (2–4 grams per day). These, along with mixed phosphate salts (3 grams daily), not only help you add more lean muscle to your body, but also may help to prevent thyroid downregulation in response to reduced-calorie diets. Consume green tea and oolong tea in place of coffee and soft drinks.

Also Consider

- Additional antioxidant nutrients.

- Digestive aids.

- Thermogenic aids for those not suffering from nervousness or related conditions.

- Other supplements geared to body type, living habits, and special circumstances.

For further information on special healing herbs and nutrients and for help in dealing with specific conditions, you will find the following books very useful:

Balch, Phyllis A., and James F. Balch. *Prescription for Nutritional Healing.* 3rd edition. Avery, 2000.

Garrison, Robert H., and Elizabeth Somer. *The Nutrition Desk Reference.* 2nd edition. Keats, 1990.

Gittleman, Ann Louise. *The Fat Flush Plan.* McGraw-Hill, 2002.

Mills, Simon Y. *Out of the Earth.* Viking, 1991.

Murray, Michael, and Joseph Pizzorno. *Encyclopedia of Natural Medicine.* 2nd edition. Prima, 1998.

Rolls, Barbara, and Robert A. Barnett. *The Volumetrics Weight-Control Plan.* HarperCollins, 2000.

Teeguarden, Ron. *Chinese Tonic Herbs.* Japan Publications, 1984.

Werbach, Melvyn R., M.D. *Healing Through Nutrition.* Harper Collins, 1993.

Werbach, Melvyn R., M.D. *Nutritional Influences on Illness.* 2nd edition. Third Line Press, 1993.

CHAPTER 4

Food Factors

A nti-fat nutrients can help you lose weight without changing your diet or increasing your activity level. However, your results will be far greater if you include regular exercise and make important dietary modifications a part of your total weight-control lifestyle. This chapter explores food and nutrition and offers some dietary practices that will help you feel great and facilitate healthful weight loss.

NUTRITION MADE EASY

Good nutrition is based on supplying yourself every day with more than forty essential nutrients. Throughout the ages this has been accomplished by the consumption of foods from the following food categories.

Animal Foods	Plant Foods
Meats	Grains
Dairy	Vegetables and seaweeds
Eggs	Beans and legumes
	Nuts and seeds
	Fruits

Although it may be possible to receive all the nutrients you need from a limited food selection, it is more enjoyable, convenient, and probably more healthful to include foods from all the food categories.

Go anywhere in the world and you will find cultures eating foods from all of the categories, perhaps with a favorite staple within each category. For example, people in the western hemisphere emphasize wheat within the grain category, whereas people in the eastern hemisphere emphasize rice. One good reason to consume a variety of foods is that a monotonous diet has been implicated in the development of food allergies.

Controversy continues with regard to the roles of fats and protein in the diet. These issues are discussed at length in Chapters 5 and 6. An increase in the consumption of fresh fruits and especially vegetables and a reduction in salt and sugar intake is recommended by most authorities.

THE DIETING DILEMMA

Most diets fail because they depend primarily upon reducing the number of calories consumed. Yet research proves that low-calorie diets are not the solution to lasting weight loss. Almost every dieter knows from experience that restricting calories very quickly reduces energy levels despite the initial weight loss common with low-calorie diets. On a daily diet of even 1,000 calories, the metabolism begins to slow down within two or three days. Your resting metabolism uses 75 percent of all the calories you burn in a given twenty-four-hour period and is reduced between 10 and 20 percent on most low-calorie diets. Since your metabolism is designed to protect you against famine, your body will always defend itself against any large reduction in calories. Even starvation diets stop working after two to three weeks. With low-calorie diets, the dieter's dilemma is that he or she must cut calories to lose weight, yet cutting calories itself slows the calorie-burning process.

The weight loss on low-calorie diets consists almost entirely of water, and the rapid weight loss of the first few weeks stops when one hits a "plateau." But this is only the beginning of the dieter's problems. After a low-calorie diet, the body's base metabolism, which is the amount of energy produced at rest, will remain depressed for several months. Then comes the "yo-yo" or rebound effect as the pounds return—with a vengeance! Low-calorie diets in reality promote fat storage, not fat burning.

FIVE PRINCIPLES FOR WEIGHT LOSS

This diet program will show you:

- How to turn off your body's fat-storage mechanism.
- How to turn on your body's fat-burning mechanism.
- How to increase your lean body-muscle tissue.
- How to increase your energy levels.
- How to reduce excess hunger and food cravings.
- How to keep the weight off and avoid the "yo-yo" dieting trap.

These goals can be accomplished by practicing a limited number of scientifically formulated principles. For example, the principles of food coupling—that is, the pairing of specific types of food, as well as the avoidance of pairing specific types of food, in a given meal—are designed specifically to balance and regulate the two major weight-controlling hormones of the body, glucagon and insulin, which will be discussed more fully in Chapter 5. For the moment, you should know that insulin is a storage hormone that inhibits the metabolism of fat for energy and generally reduces the metabolic rate, whereas glucagon releases sugar sources (glycogen and some amino acids) from storage in the liver so that they can be turned into blood sugar (glucose) and used for fuel.

Principle 1: Avoid fat storage by practicing proper "food coupling." (Keys to proper food coupling directly follow Principle 5.)

Fat is a concentrated source of calories with about twice as many calories per gram (9 per gram) as are found in either carbohydrates or proteins. Fat-heavy meals lack bulk, so they make it easy to consume hundreds of calories without feeling full.

When fat is eaten at the same time as simple carbohydrates, both the fat and the carbohydrates are pushed into storage. This is to say that stored fat increases, blood fat levels soar, and the body's basic blood sugar control mechanism is damaged. The "bad" coupling of fats with carbohydrates slows down your metabolism and causes you to gain weight.

To avoid weight gain, avoid all sugars and simple carbohydrates and especially avoid fat/carbohydrate couplings such as are found in fried foods, cakes and cookies, sweet rolls, candy bars, and so on. Avoid all fruit juices since these are concentrated sources of sugar. Limit whole fruits to two servings per day. Emphasize whole grains, legumes, lean proteins, and lightly cooked fresh vegetables.

Protein/carbohydrate couplings also should be kept to a minimum. Most protein foods contain fat (for example, most meats, eggs, and milk). Moreover, research indicates that protein/carbohydrate combinations may reduce the body's ability to release growth hormone (GH), a major fat-burning hormone, because of the additive effect that many proteins have on the amount of insulin released in response to carbohydrates.

Sugars and other refined carbohydrates increase the absorption of dietary fats while reducing the oxidation of fats for energy. (In ingredient lists, sugars are easy to spot; they are the substances ending in "ose.") All the common food sources of sugar can be reduced to a very few chemically related sugar molecules, mainly glucose, fructose, and galactose. Glucose and fructose are "simple sugars" and are called monosaccharides, "mono" meaning "one." Disaccharides ("di" meaning "two") are constructed from two sugar molecules, usually glucose and/or fructose. The common disaccharides are sucrose, lactose, and maltose. Our digestive system reduces most carbohydrates to glucose, that is, blood sugar. However, fructose is also taken up directly into the blood and into the cells. Cane sugar, which is also called sucrose, is a combination of glucose and fructose linked together. Milk sugar, or lactose, is made up of linked molecules of glucose and galactose. Grape sugar, which otherwise is called dextrose, is actually glucose. Honey consists mostly of the simple sugars glucose and fructose, but also contains sucrose, and is sweeter to the taste than table sugar. The evidence against coupling refined carbohydrates with fats is clear and unambiguous. Consider the study results outlined below.

- Taken in a milk shake, fructose (30 grams) increased postprandial lipemia (that is, increase in blood fats following meals) by 37 percent compared with control; glucose (17.5 grams) increased postprandial lipemia by 59 percent.[1]

- In Syndrome X (insulin-resistant) subjects (BMI of 30), glucose consumption (50 grams) led to a 15.9 percent greater glycemic response and a 30.9 percent greater insulin response than did fructose consumption (50 grams). In Syndrome X subjects, therefore, sugars that require an insulin response can lead both to elevated blood sugar and to an elevated insulin level. This data would appear to indicate that fructose, which largely bypasses the insulin response, is a "good" sugar. However, fructose does even more to prevent the burning of fat for energy than does glucose, as the next point indicates.

- On an energy-balanced diet in these same Syndrome X subjects, fructose compared with glucose increased carbohydrate oxidation by 31 percent, but decreased fat oxidation by 39 percent. Thus fructose consumption, even more so than the consumption of other sugar sources, makes burning stored fat for energy more difficult.[2]

- Low-fat, high-carbohydrate diets in Syndrome X individuals reduce levels of HDL cholesterol (the "good" cholesterol) and increase triacylglycerol concentrations.[3]

Note: Triacylglycerol (as in triacylglycerol-rich lipoproteins) is a blood fat component related to triglycerides. Triacylglycerols tend to be elevated in the blood after meals, are especially high in diabetics and those with Syndrome X, and are probably more contributory to atherosclerosis than all the usually monitored blood fractions of LDL cholesterol taken together.

Principle 2: Turn on your metabolism naturally with the proper food choices. Burn stored fat for energy and for body heat.
Some foods burn "hotter" than others; that is, they cause your body to expend more calories for heat, encourage activity, and are not as readily stored. Proteins and complex carbohydrates are "hot" burners. They are not easily stored as fat and they tell your body it has plenty of fuel, so it is all right to go ahead and spend energy. This explains the "thermic" or heat-producing effect of eating a meal; it "turns on" your metabolism.

As many will know, sugars (mono- and disaccharides) and sugar sources, such as all fruit juices, are simple carbohydrates. Because food processing tends to increase the rate at which starches and other carbohydrates are turned into glucose and released into the bloodstream, white flour and other processed grain products, cereals, and even many canned items must be treated as sources of simple carbohydrates. Whole grains, whole-grain products, and nearly all vegetables can be considered sources of complex carbohydrates. Whole fruit, because of its fiber content, is more "complex" than its fruit juice.

For especially energizing meals, couple lean proteins (such as fish, skinless chicken, lean beef or lamb, and tofu) with a variety of non-starchy vegetables. If a meal contains no concentrated carbohydrates (no breads, grains, potatoes, and so on), you need not be particularly concerned about its fat content. Couple complex carbohydrates with vegetables (and a small amount of lean protein) for satisfying and more bulky meals.

Principle 3: Exercise to increase your metabolic efficiency and to train your body to burn stored fat for energy.
Exercise burns calories, but the greatest benefit comes after the exercise has ended. If you walk briskly for a mere thirty minutes per day, you will increase your calorie burning for the entire twenty-four-hour period. Adding a moderate amount of upper-body exercise or weight lifting will improve your energy expenditure even more by adding calorie-burning lean muscle tissue to your body. For weight loss, plan on walking briskly for at least thirty minutes every day. This is best done either before or

after breakfast. A walk early in the day while the body's temperature is still rising will invigorate you for the rest of the day. The second best time for a walk is after your last meal of the day. Walking after meals is a particularly good practice for diabetics and for those genetically prone to developing diabetes.

Principle 4: Add fiber to your diet, and avoid refined and processed foods.
Fiber slows down food consumption so that your body has a chance to signal that you have eaten enough. It adds bulk to the meal to give you a feeling of satisfaction at having eaten. It slows the blood sugar increase that follows any meal. Fiber carries waste products from the body, and, especially if it comes from lightly cooked vegetables, it supplies important minerals and antioxidants. Try to vary your fiber sources. Avoid too much scratchy wheat bran, but add to your menu grains, such as oats and barley, and starchy vegetables, such as sweet potatoes and yams (without added butter and sugar). Try to eliminate refined and processed foods from your diet. Eliminate all commercial canned and frozen foods—these often contain hidden fats and sugars.

Principle 5: Use anti-fat nutrients and thermogenic enhancers.
Many individuals who are overweight find that they need a little help to "jump start" their ability to burn fat. See the basic program given in Chapter 3 for guidance in designing your own anti-fat nutrient program.

KEYS TO FOOD COUPLING FOR WEIGHT CONTROL

The Anti-Fat Nutrient Weight-Loss Program advocates a non-calorie-restricted diet based upon a moderate and sustainable eating pattern. What you eat, when you eat it, and which foods you eat together are far more important than the number of calories you consume. Follow these three simple keys:

KEY #1: Avoid Foods That Combine Fats with Simple Carbohydrates

First of all, avoid all sugars. Eat no more than two servings of fruit a day and drink no fruit juices. Also limit protein/carbohydrate combinations.

This is the most important part of your diet: Avoid foods that contain fat and simple carbohydrate combinations. These include French fries, buttered breads, cakes, cookies, candies, most bakery products, canned and frozen foods with added corn syrup or fructose, milk shakes, ice cream, most fast foods, packaged corn and potato chips, peanut butter sandwiches, most packaged snack foods, and so on. Simple sugars are found in fruit juices, soft drinks, most prepared breakfast cereals, many canned and frozen foods, and most so-called diet powders and diet drinks. Eat unprocessed and unrefined foods whenever possible. A small amount of olive oil used in pasta sauces and in cooking is allowable.

KEY #2: Couple Proteins with Vegetables

Trim the visible fats from meats, but do not attempt to make protein meals "fat free." You can eat unlimited amounts of non-starchy (primarily green) vegetables and limited amounts of starchy vegetables in protein-containing meals. Small amounts ($1/4$ cup) of all nuts (raw), except peanuts, can be eaten.

Proteins include, in order of preference, fish, turkey, chicken, other poultry, lamb, beef, pork, eggs, and cheese. Beans and other legumes are better considered as complex carbohydrates than as proteins. Milk interferes with the digestion of other proteins and should be taken alone. Unrestricted vegetables include asparagus, green beans, broccoli, cabbage, cauliflower, celery, cilantro, kale, mustard and other "greens," green and red peppers, scallions, spinach, and zucchini; these are best lightly steamed but may be sautéed in a little olive oil. Starchy vegetables, including beets, carrots, corn, green peas, pumpkin, and winter squashes, should be limited to half a cup in any meal containing fats.

KEY #3: Couple Complex Carbohydrates and Starches with Vegetables

Avoid fats and limit protein (less than $1/4$ cup) in carbohydrate-containing meals. Small amounts ($1/4$ cup) of all nuts (raw), except peanuts, can be eaten. Try to use natural insulin-potentiating spices, such as bay leaf or curry, at meals that include rice or potatoes.

Complex carbohydrates include whole-grain wheat, corn, barley, oats, millet, brown rice, buckwheat, amaranth, and quiona. Excellent non-grain starches are potatoes, sweet potatoes, yams, and most beans and other legumes. At meals, these complex carbohydrates and starches can be eaten in moderate quantities, combined with vegetables that can be eaten in unlimited quantities. Small amounts of olive oil used in pasta sauces and in cooking are allowable.

Food-Coupling Do's and Don'ts

Do	Don't
Fat-Burning Couplings	**Fat-Storing Couplings**
protein (4–6 oz) + green vegetables (limit starchy vegetables to ½ cup)	protein + carbohydrates
carbohydrates* + all vegetables**	fats + carbohydrates
starches* + all vegetables**	fats + starches
carbohydrates* + fruits***	proteins/fats + fruits

*Complex carbohydrates and starches: whole grains, whole-wheat pastas and breads, beans and legumes, potatoes, sweet potatoes, and yams.

**Includes starchy and high-carbohydrate vegetables: corn, beets, green peas, lima beans, snow peas, and winter squashes.

***Exclude melons: Melons should be eaten alone.

Most dieters find that increasing the amount of protein in their diets improves both energy and appetite control. Protein goes well with complex carbohydrates and vegetables. If you make fish your preferred source of protein, rather than red meat, you will enjoy the extra benefits of essential oils. Encourage maximum weight loss by having two protein-based meals and one carbohydrate-based meal per day. Remember to integrate the Anti-Fat Nutrient Weight-Loss Program in Chapter 3 with the three keys to food coupling above.

TIPS FOR WEIGHT LOSS

Once you grasp the keys to successful food coupling, and are supplementing your diet with the nutrient regimen described in the Core Program in Chapter 3, you will be well on your way to reducing unwanted body fat. This section contains some hints to help you continue on the path to greater health and vitality.

Never Skip Breakfast

Your first meal tends to set the tone for the rest of the day, and the next meal, in terms of importance, is lunch. Studies typically find that those of us who habitually consume at least half of our total daily calories in our first two meals stay slimmer and trimmer. Skipping breakfast triggers the "starvation response," slows your metabolism, and may contribute to calories being stored as fat. Substituting a cup of coffee and a sweet roll for breakfast is almost as bad as not eating. Eat early to keep your energy levels up during the day, but try not to eat within three hours of bedtime (those calories mostly end up stored as fat). Eating very late in the day also makes it more difficult to wake up in the morning.

Eat Foods High in Fiber

Dieters who eat high-fiber foods have been shown to lose more weight than those not eating as much fiber. Individuals who stay slim average 50 percent more fiber in their diets than do those who are heavier. Whole fruits, vegetables, legumes, whole grains, and other high-fiber foods slow the release of sugars into the bloodstream and thus help to give you more even, steady levels of energy. Also, fiber is bulky and helps us to feel more satisfied with fewer calories at meals. The fiber in vegetables is more easily digested if lightly cooked.

Avoid Refined Foods and Sugars, Limit Fruit Juices

Simple carbohydrates lead to fat storage because they interfere with the body's ability to burn fat. Refined and processed foods are often loaded with salt, sugar, and fat. Processing and overcooking makes most foods, even complex carbohydrates, act like sugar in the body. Fruit juices and overly ripe fruit or very sweet fruits also act like sugar in the body. Favor items such as whole oranges, apples, cherries, berries, and peaches. However, no more than two whole fruits should be eaten daily. Replace wheat breads with whole rye, spelt, barley, oat, and other breads whenever possible. Avoid more than occasional consumption of soft drinks, including so-called diet drinks. Avoid caffeine unless it is specifically a part of your anti-fat nutrient program. Caffeine in excess or taken late in the day prevents sound sleep. Sound sleep in the first few hours after going to bed is important for the proper functioning of the body's hormonal system.

Drink More Water

Just as starving yourself triggers the "starvation response," not drinking enough water causes the body to retain fluid. Drinking plenty of water also helps the body to dispose of toxins. Drink eight to ten glasses of pure water every day. Coffee, tea, and soft drinks are not good substitutes for water because they may act as diuretics, contain sugars, or otherwise fail to be good sources for rehydration.

Avoid Processed Fats and Oils

Eat the oils suggested in the Core Program, but avoid margarine and other processed or artificially hardened oils. Eliminate fried foods, cookies, pastries, and prepared salad dressings. For cooking, use extra virgin olive oil. For salad dressings, use cold-pressed olive, walnut, canola, or sunflower-seed oil in small amounts with lemon juice.

Limit Alcohol

The typical American diet obtains as much as 10 percent of its calories from alcohol. Keep drinks that contain alcohol to no more than two per day. Alcohol, if consumed, should be combined with meals rather than consumed alone or before meals.

Make Only Moderate Changes in Your Total Daily Caloric Intake

The infamous "yo-yo" pattern of weight loss and regain is caused by excessive calorie cutting for rapid weight loss. Aim for steady and sustained weight loss, instead. If you count calories, cut back to 90 percent of the calories that you would consume without dieting. If you find yourself "binging," you may be cutting your food intake too drastically.

Eat Slowly and Deliberately, Eat Smaller Meals

Eating too quickly or eating in front of the TV encourages weight gain. Eating very large meals makes digestion more difficult, makes you sluggish, and encourages excessive insulin response. If you feel hungry during the day, snack on hard vegetables (for example, carrots or celery) or, as a second choice, eat a serving of a hard fruit (for example, a hard apple) or a cup of vegetable soup, rather than allowing yourself to become too hungry. This way, you will not overeat at the next meal.

Take a Good Multivitamin and Mineral Supplement

Vitamin and mineral deficiencies can trigger the "starvation response." Minerals such as chromium are important in the body's regulation of carbohydrate and fat metabolism.

Exercise Daily

A good twenty- to thirty-minute walk is a great way to get into an exercise routine. Walking early in the day helps the body to "wake up." Walking more than once per day can improve your rate of weight loss. Exercise is important primarily for training your body to release and burn fats for energy. Weight training to add lean muscle tissue can encourage your body to burn calories.

Super Tip for Meals

If you follow some or all of the tips above, you will certainly witness the loss of unwanted pounds. However, we have saved for last the tip that will enable you to rein in your ravenous impulses at mealtimes, allowing you to feel satisfied without filling up with empty calories.

For both lunch and supper, have a bowl of clear or vegetable (not cream) soup as the first course in place of salad. If you wish, a small salad can be eaten alongside the main course instead—that is, unless a salad, such as a chef's salad, itself is the main course. Most people will find that their digestion of protein (beef, fish, chicken, tofu, etc.) will be improved if they do not start the meal with a large serving of raw vegetables.

Next, make sure that one-half—or even two-thirds—of your plate is covered with the lightly cooked vegetable of your choice (salad does not count here, and corn and carrots are counted as carbohydrates). Always eat this vegetable serving, which should be at least 2 cups of vegetables. Eat a bit of protein before eating any carbohydrate in the main meal. It is as simple as that. Once weight loss has been achieved, the program can be expanded to include a piece of whole fruit as dessert after meals.

CHAPTER 5

The End of Dieting

We all know famous personalities, such as Oprah Winfrey, who heroically and publicly have lost a great deal of weight on this or that special diet, only to regain the lost pounds month by month. Recently the National Instituts of Health estimated that nearly 90 percent of dieters regain all or most of their lost weight within five years, then repeat the cycle of diet and weight gain once again. A large and thriving industry, which sells billions of dollars a year in diet products and services, has emerged to take advantage of the difficulties and the frustration that many face when they attempt to lose weight. The aim of this book is to help its readers avoid both the desperation and the relapse so typical of dieting, and to do so without costing the hundreds of dollars charged by various special programs and clinics.

Any number of dieters find themselves caught in this trap of using a crash diet to lose weight, only to have the pounds return with a vengeance and refuse to come off a second time. Others lose weight, seemingly successfully, yet when they look in the mirror they still do not like what they see. There are at least five reasons for these disappointing results of good intentions and considerable effort. Three of these reasons are physiological and two are psychological, but quite real. To begin with the physiological issues, these include diet-induced hypothyroidism (low thyroid function) and other diet-induced metabolic imbalances, the loss of lean tissues, and the ramifications of metabolic individuality. Let's take a look at this last issue first. . . .

THE THREE METABOLIC BODY TYPES AND FAT METABOLISM

Before beginning any program for personal transformation, it is a good idea to consider why this change is desirable and just what it is that you want to achieve. Losing weight is no exception to this rule. Good reasons include considerations such as health, beauty, and athletic performance. Bad reasons often mimic good ones, but usually bad reasons are rooted in unrealistic expectations and other psychological factors, rather than in one's physiology. One of the most common unrealistic expectations concerns appearance. TV and the press bombard us with images of "ideal" bodies, images of models and athletes, and so forth, but these are images that represent the natural body types of only a small percentage of the population—they are not most of us. Finding one's ideal weight means finding a healthful and sustainable weight that fits one's own metabolic individuality.

Physiologists commonly divide us into three general body types: ectomorphs, mesomorphs, and endomorphs. These body types are inherited, although they can be influenced by diet and activities during the first two decades of life. Body types are rough guides to individual metabolic rates and to fat metabolism. It is not possible for us to change our body types, and therefore it is unrealistic to expect any diet or exercise program to accomplish this feat. Dieters should discover what is realistic for their own body types and likewise discover the strengths that are the special virtues of each type. This is a much better approach than for all of us to attempt to be the same "ideal" person.

Ectomorphs

The ectomorphs are naturally slender individuals who find it difficult to gain weight no matter how much they eat. Their metabolisms are fast burning and their ability to convert food to fat is limited. Often they have great difficulty putting on muscle tissue, as well. These "thin no matter how much they eat" types are often the envy of their heavier cousins, but this attitude is very much a product of the plenty that characterizes food sources for most Americans. Historically, the ability to gain weight when food was plentiful was a survival mechanism. It defended against periods of famine and it insulated the body against cold. These facts can be seen geographically in the populations of Europe. There is a crude gradient that runs from the warmer and more temperate West and South (for example, England, France, and Spain) to the generally colder East (Russia). Naturally occurring body fat is a higher percentage of total body weight in the East than in the West, and this inherited physiology reflects in part the harsher climate and the more unstable food supply as one

moves eastward. Being an ectomorph may be great if you want to be a bas-
ketball star or a willowy fashion model, but it is not so good if you want
to survive a winter in Siberia.

Can ectomorphs become obese? Yes, they certainly can. Typical ecto-
morphic cases of obesity may have been pencil thin in their early twenties or even later, but thereafter they gain weight rapidly. Ectomorphs are
more prone than other body types to psychological factors, such as nervousness, worry, anxiety, and fear. To calm their nerves they may overeat
and, especially, they may indulge in sugars and simple carbohydrates
since these foods tend to encourage the production of the calming neurochemical serotonin in the brain. Also, feelings of security or stability
may come with the added weight. For these nervous types, calorie restriction is likely not the primary answer to weight problems. Rather, calming
the excess nervousness, whatever its source, is the better solution. Whole
grains and starchy vegetables can help calm the nerves without encouraging excess pounds, and various herbs and moderate exercise can be
tried to reduce hyperactivity. This body type will also benefit from regular schedules for activities and meals.

Mesomorphs

Mesomorphs are your typical athletic types. They tend to be large-boned,
more heavily muscled, and lean in their earlier years. Many of our cham-
pion bodybuilders are of this type, as, again, are many fashion models and
actresses. Arnold Schwarzenegger and Jane Fonda come immediately to
mind. Gifted with physical prowess in their early and middle years, mesomorphs are likely to begin to put on weight in later life as they slow down
metabolically (we all do) and cease to be as active, yet continue to eat
much the same diet as they had in their youth because they have much
the same appetite. Some of those most dissatisfied with their bodies after,
say, age forty, are mesomorphs.

Weight gain in mesomorphs is most commonly the result of simple
overconsumption. The appetite is good, so eating is satisfying in itself. The
weight gained by mesomorphs often is much "firmer" than is that gained
by ectomorphs, for the mesomorphs continue to have more muscle.
Mesomorphs also like the feeling of power and stimulation given to them
by red meats and other concentrated proteins, and also by spicy and fatty
dishes that activate the liver. However, in the usual American cuisine, red
meats contain lots of fats as well as proteins, and all these dishes are

often combined with one or more relatively simple carbohydrate. Such combinations tend to have highly undesirable effects upon insulin production, and this leads to fat storage. Finally, inasmuch as excess protein intake makes many people more aggressive, mesomorphs, who do not usually need any additional drive or aggression, tend to consume beer and other alcoholic beverages "to relax." Alcohol itself has many calories and it also interferes with the metabolism of fat. Neither of these qualities is useful for someone who is overweight.

As a rule, of our three body types, it is the mesomorphs who can most easily regain their proper proportions simply by reining in the consumption of excess calories *if their weight gain has not gone on for too long or become too excessive.* True obesity, the gain of weight to something above 20 percent of one's ideal weight, tends to derange the metabolism. Whether this is ascribed to the body's having established a new "set point" (either a brain or a fat-cell-mediated level of body weight) or to other mechanisms, once the derangement has taken place, it requires considerable effort to correct.

Endomorphs

The endomorphs are individuals who put on weight easily and do not shed it readily. They likely have been what they consider "heavy" for most of their lives. If not too excessively self-conscious about their weight, these individuals tend to be somewhat more relaxed and calmer than the first two types. If their weight is brought into a balance appropriate for their body type, these individuals also tend to have considerable physical endurance and mental staying power. Famous opera singers notoriously have endomorphic characteristics, but so did the great philosophers St. Thomas Aquinas and David Hume. Many professional football players display large degrees of endomorphy, but so does Marlon Brando. And what woman is not envious of the hair, eyes, and complexion of Elizabeth Taylor, who, again, has some strong endomorphic traits?

Endomorphic obesity often is related to a slow metabolism. This may be the result of inadequate thyroid production or of other hormonal conditions; it may be the result of the simple tendency toward inactivity; or it may be the consequence of the desire to have comfort, such as good food. The kidneys may be slow and there may be a tendency toward water retention for any number of reasons. In any event, this body type does well by avoiding all simple carbohydrates and also excess salt. Since there is already a tendency to store excess calories as fats, endomorphs do well to restrict all sources of concentrated calories. Bulky foods, such as raw and cooked vegetables, whole grains and beans, and so on, are good choices, as are foods that increase thermogenesis. Aerobic exercise to speed up the metabolism is a great idea; excess sleep and naps probably should be avoided. More especially, the amount of time spent in front of the television should be strictly controlled. TV watching has been shown to dramatically lower basal metabolic rates for many individuals, and the amount of time spent in front of the television is the second best predictor of obesity known![1]

These three body types respond differently to the same diets, and even at their ideal weights they will never look the same. And why should they? Most of us have bodies that are combinations of ectomorphy, mesomorphy, and endomorphy in varying degrees. Each of us can obtain our own ideal weight, but it must match the body we have.

The ectomorph/mesomorph/endomorph taxonomy is a simple one commonly used, but it is not the only one available. In the last decade, Dr. Elliot D. Abravanel wrote two books based upon the notion that each of us has a dominant hormonal system. During the same period Dr. Jeffrey Bland, a well-published author of books on nutrition, put forward his diet based upon the individual's efficiency at metabolizing fats, carbohydrates, and proteins. Yet another taxonomy was published recently by Dr. Deepak Chopra, this one based upon Ayurveda, the ancient Indian medical system of classification and treatment. The interested reader might want to consult these authors for fuller treatments of the notion of individual body types.[2] Not surprisingly, there tends to be a large degree of overlap among the various systems used to classify physiological types. The suggestions given above are by no means definitive, but they are useful guides for beginning the process of balancing one's own particular body type.

The usual medical definition of obesity classifies anyone who is 20 percent or more over his or her desirable weight as obese. This definition is tricky in that one's ideal weight depends upon the size and type of frame that characterizes the body. Large-boned individuals will quite naturally carry more weight than those with light bones, which is to say that ectomorphs and mesomorphs of the same age and height generally should not weigh the same. A number of charts and tables have been prepared listing desirable weights for men and women, and your family physician will likely be able to show you one or more of these. The most commonly used one was prepared for the Metropolitan Life Insurance Company in 1959. Those either far below or far above the listed weights are thought to be at considerable additional risk of various illnesses, and the 20 percent figure for medically defining obesity was derived from statistics that indicate it is only at this point that the death rate begins markedly to exceed normal. That is, the mortality rate at this point climbs for those not *already* suffering from high blood pressure, high blood lipids, or diabetes, all conditions which themselves are usually associated with excess weight. Some more cautious medical authorities define obesity as anything above 10 percent of one's desirable weight.

Another way of defining ideal weight is to use the percentage of adult weight that is devoted to fat. One source (*The Physician and Sportsmedicine,* April 1986) considers men obese if this percentage is above 25 percent, and women obese if it is above 30 percent. The body-fat percentage associated with optimal health for men can range from 10 to 25 percent, and for women, from 18 to 30 percent.

Neither of these ways of determining ideal weight is without its critics, and there is little agreement over how much damage is inflicted on one's health by being *moderately* overweight. As with the case of body-type variations, genetic background appears to be very important in determining just how much risk a few extra pounds pose to health. Discovering whether you qualify as obese under an accepted medical definition will probably require the help of a doctor.[3] In 1983 roughly 40 million Americans were estimated to be obese in the medical sense, and another 40 million were probably above their desirable weights; two-thirds of these individuals were over the age of forty. There is a great deal of evidence that genetics plays a role in determining adult weight.[4] Nevertheless, it is likely that excess weight for most "heavy" individuals is the result of inadequate exercise, faulty diet, or related reasons.

Since the majority of readers no doubt already are aware that obesity brings health risks, the point will not be belabored here. Virtually all those involved medically in the care of the overweight, no matter their other differences, agree on a long list of complaints either directly or indirectly linked to excess weight. This list includes most or all of the following: increased risk of cardiovascular disease, diabetes, high blood pressure, stroke, and diseases of the blood vessels, gallbladder, kidneys, and liver. Fortunately, many of these conditions can be stabilized or even improved through the loss of excess weight.

This list of ailments is a bit frightening, and it should be. More disturbing, however, is the fact that dieting itself often greatly worsens a bad situation. Crash diets place extreme stress on the body. The rapid weight gain that usually follows fad diets is more damaging in that it causes elevation of unwanted blood lipids, increased rates of plaque deposits on artery walls, and other damage to the body. The Framingham Study of heart disease indicated that those who were obese at the start of the study and who lost 10 percent of their body weight cut their chances of heart disease by some 20 percent. However, if they gained back those same pounds, their risk rate jumped 30 percent; that is, it became higher than it would have been had they never dieted.[5]

Nevertheless, the good news from the Framingham Study is that a 10 percent reduction of body weight for those who at the start were clinically obese is significant if maintained. Every extra pound above the ideal is associated with a 2 percent increase in mortality rates, primarily from heart disease and cancer.[6] Indeed, the connection between weight and mortality is so strong that critics of American medical dietary recommendations for controlling blood cholesterol levels through changes in diet have often noted that unless the obese subjects lost weight, changing the composition of the diet to radically reduce saturated-fat consumption generally had little or no significant effect on blood lipid levels, and certainly no effect on mortality rates.[7]

YOUR IDEAL WEIGHT

Your ideal weight, as has been indicated already, depends upon a number of factors. However, the two most important of these are the size and density of your bones, and the ratio of lean tissue to fat stores. Weight charts have difficulty in accurately placing individuals by bone weight, relying on visible features; for example, they describe people as having small, medium, and large frames.

Likewise, the ratio of lean to fat tissue is best measured medically by the displacement of water in an underwater weight test to yield the body's specific gravity. Often the first stage of weight gain involves no gain of weight at all, but rather the loss of muscle tissue and its displacement by adipose tissue. This shows up as a change in the specific gravity of the body. Only after the metabolism has begun to slow down because of the loss of energy-burning muscle does the individual begin to markedly put on weight and then find this weight difficult to remove. The moral is that scale weight taken by itself is less significant than is normally assumed.

Nevertheless, studies have shown that dieters are more successful by far in achieving a desirable weight, and in maintaining that weight, if they have an ideal weight clearly in mind. Therefore, readers might try this suggestion from *The Endocrine Control Diet:* "One rule of thumb that has been used for determining ideal body weight for men is 106 pounds for the first 5 feet of height and 6 pounds for each inch after 5 feet, plus or minus 10 percent according to frame size. The rule for women is 100 pounds for the first 5 feet, and 5 pounds per inch thereafter, with the same adjustment for frame size."[8] For the sake of comparison, consider that the so-called ideal weight for successful endurance runners has been estimated to be twice their height in inches, that is, a male runner who is 5 feet 10 inches, or 70 inches tall, should weigh 140 pounds.[9]

WHY DIETS DON'T WORK

The physiological reasons for diet failure apply to pretty much everyone who diets, and virtually every professional in the field of weight loss acknowledges their impact. As a general rule, diets that take off more than 2 pounds per week remove primarily water and/or lean tissue from the body. Diets based on diuretics ("water pills") do this directly, but much the same effect is achieved by most (but not all) low-carbohydrate diets. For example, many high-protein diets often work for a period of time because protein is an inefficient source of energy that floods the bloodstream with nitrogen byproducts as it is broken down to yield calories. Ammonia and urea are toxic to the body. They are known to be hard on the liver and even harder on the kidneys. Needless to say, these waste products do not make the dieter feel better. People lose weight rapidly on low-carbohydrate diets mostly due to a loss of water as the kidneys draw moisture from the tissues in order to flush protein waste products from the body. This is to say that your body chooses the lesser of evils, forfeiting necessary hydration to rid itself of toxins. However, as soon as the diet ends, the desiccated tissues are quickly rehydrated and the "lost" weight is regained.

Diets that are extremely low in calories—no matter how well balanced in terms of quality proteins, vitamins, electrolytes, and so forth—ultimately are counterproductive because they convince the body that it is starving, so it shuts down to conserve energy. The abrupt restriction of calories leads to diminished thyroid activity within as few as two days. This fact is significant because one of the main stimulants of energy consumption and of general physical activity is the thyroid hormone. The thyroid also is very important for thermogenesis, the production of body heat, and dieters usually should be aiming to increase this process. Yet to guard against the seeming starvation of crash diets, the body shuts down thyroid production to conserve energy, and depression of thyroid activity in turn is linked to the reduction of fat mobilization and to an increase in fat storage. The results are that the dieter feels tired and the number of calories burned daily actually declines. Similarly, since the body is trying to prevent starvation, it begins primarily to use up those tissues that burn calories, that is, the body's lean muscle tissues—rather than the fat the dieter wants to lose. The body's logic is simple: reduce the calorie-burning lean tissues and you reduce the danger of starvation. If this were not bad enough, the energy inefficiency and the sheer toxicity of many diets, through yet other mechanisms, again may cause the loss of lean tissues, including those of the heart.

To be sure, there are specially designed very-low-calorie, high-protein diets that aim to spare the lean tissues while encouraging moderate *ketosis,* the burning of the body's fat stores for fuel. However, even the best of such diets run up against the body's defense mechanisms intended to prevent starvation. Moreover, since dieters can achieve the same mild ketosis in very-low-carbohydrate, high-protein diets without expensive diet powders or liquids and without an extreme restriction of calories, the usefulness of even the best of the very-low-calorie, high-protein diets is questionable. This is not to say that well-designed very-low-calorie diets that spare proteins cannot help one lose weight *in the short term*—clinically they often have been shown to lead to significant weight loss—but only to warn that they may not be the best way to go and that the weight lost through such diets will likely come back.

In brief, during a crash diet, the body defends itself against what it perceives as starvation by cannibalizing the muscle tissue that uses up calories and thus threatens survival under famine conditions. At the same time the depression of thyroid production makes it harder for the body to burn fats. Indeed, as much as 30 percent of the weight lost during a typical crash diet is from muscle loss. Moreover, the body's energy-conservation measures can be so effective that some people cannot lose weight even consuming only 750 calories a day, which is about one-third of a normal daily consumption of calories![10]

WEIGHT LOSS IS EASY—FAT LOSS IS NOT

Now for some slightly more technical explanations of what happens on crash diets. The first physiological change brought on by a crash diet is the loss of lean tissue, and this loss means that the dieter's entire metabolism slows down. Lean tissue burns calories twenty-four hours a day, and it is the muscle-to-fat ratio that often is most important in determining how well the body handles calories. The loss of lean tissue results in the lasting reduction of what is called the basal metabolic rate (BMR), the rate at which the resting body normally uses energy, whereas an increase in the muscle-to-fat ratio heightens the BMR.[11] Therefore, after the crash diet ends, the body needs fewer calories to sustain itself, and even on a restricted maintenance diet the pounds will slowly return. Likewise, dieters may find that they seem to have permanently lost a certain amount of energy and perhaps, as well, that they do not respond properly to colder temperatures by increasing body warmth. And, of course, fat reserves, which do not burn calories, actually have become a larger proportion of all the body's tissues. When the disappointed dieters go back on their former diet, they find it much harder to lose the weight a second time since their metabolism has slowed down. The weight comes back more quickly, and often they gain even more weight. J. S. Stern and others in the article "Weighing the Options: Criteria for Evaluating Weight-Management Programs" explain: "those who complete weight-loss programs lose approximately 10 percent of their body weight, only to regain two-thirds of it back within one year and almost all of it back within five years."[12]

The second physiological change caused by crash diets is a bit more subtle than the first, but every bit as detrimental. When the body is presented with what seems to be starvation, it activates a number of hormones involved in fat storage while reducing the production of hormones that cause the body to burn fat for energy. The reduction in catabolic thyroid activity has already been mentioned. Other hormones, such as insulin and an enzyme called lipoprotein lipase (LPL), are anabolic in nature. Together these anabolic hormones and changes cause the body to begin to store food as fat, even when only a very few calories are consumed. (See "Hypothyroidism, Liver Function, and Brown Fat" later in this chapter.) Once hormones such as LPL in fatty tissues have been activated for any length of time under quasi-famine conditions, it is very hard to convince the body to turn them off again. Moreover, fat storage may begin even before the diet actually has ended. On some high-protein diets the body can turn the excess protein into enough sugar so that the unused portion is stored by insulin as fat. As the dieter returns to a normal number of calories after the diet, the anabolic hormones continue to conserve energy and to store calories. After the diet is over, the unfortunate dieter may put on 10 pounds before the regulatory mechanisms quiet and return to something approaching their normal ranges. With successive crash diets, the body finds it easier to turn on energy-sparing hormones and more difficult to turn them off.[13] One reason that dieters who exercise consistently are more successful is that, unlike fat cells, muscle cells use LPL to release fats from blood triglycerides for fuel. Studies show that the detraining of athletes results in a decrease in muscle LPL, whereas adipose-tissue LPL increases. This decrease in muscle LPL, coupled with an increase in adipose LPL, yields a condition favoring fat storage in adipose tissues.[14]

The third physiological limitation of most diets is that they fail to take into account metabolic individuality; therefore, they usually fail to address the actual causes of unwanted weight gain. Some people gain weight because they are inactive, some because of the combinations of foods in their diets, still others because of faulty regulatory mechanisms. It is highly unlikely that all these different individuals can be helped by using exactly the same diet, and the sources of their problems are not the same. (See "The Three Metabolic Body Types and Fat Metabolism" on page 104.)

Aside from the severe physiological drawbacks of the usual crash diets, there are psychological drawbacks as well. For one, the dieter wants fat loss, not just weight loss. To get the proper "look," the desired shapeliness of the body, the body's fat must be where it belongs, that is, mainly between the skin and the muscle. Excess fat commonly is spread into other tissues. When this fat is lost, and much muscle along with it, the dieter still looks and feels flabby even though she or he may now be at the weight given as ideal on the charts. The diet has done nothing to improve the tone of the muscles or the shape of the body. As a result, the dieter feels unsatisfied even after having lost a great deal of weight.

A second psychological drawback of most diets is that they do not address the cravings that cause many people to overeat or to eat the wrong foods. These cravings themselves often have a basis in physiology or even in brain biochemistry, so they seldom are "all in one's head." But regardless of how the cravings are defined, a brief look at a few of them will show why diets rarely are the answer to the mischief such cravings cause. Surveys have shown that half of all respondents admit that they tend to use food as an answer to depression. Significantly, solace is not sought in protein foods, for which consumption remains largely steady under a variety of circumstances, but in fats, sweets, and other carbohydrates. In one poll done for the *Wall Street Journal,* ice cream and chocolate bars topped the list of mood-dependent food choices, followed in order by pizza, beer, soft drinks, hot soup, peanut butter, and hamburgers.

Sometimes cravings are rooted in memories of home or happy times; sometimes they are rooted in desires to be "bad" or to punish oneself or others. Yet brain chemistry may supply better answers than simple memory. Judith Wurtman, a nutritional chemist at MIT, argues that carbohydrates tend to calm us and to provide energy while relieving depression. Reactions vary with individuals, but the calming response appears to be related to the ability of carbohydrates to increase the presence of the neurotransmitter serotonin in the brain, while at the same time the increase in blood sugar temporarily elevates mood in those with uneven blood sugar control. (Proteins, in contrast to carbohydrates, tend to stimulate the central nervous system and thus make us more active.)

Adam Drewnowski of the University of Michigan suggests that the neurochemical link may be even stronger. Food cravings in some people may alter the level of endorphins, naturally occurring, potent mood-altering brain chemicals similar to narcotics in their effects. Drewnowski's research indicates that many food cravings can be blocked by the drug naloxone, which, in clinical settings, sometimes is employed to ease opiate cravings.[15]

The point is that most diets attempt to reduce only the consequence of food cravings, that is, excess weight. These diets do nothing to reduce the cravings themselves nor to address their causes. Thus, just as these diets, for physiological reasons, fail to keep weight off (that is, they do not prevent the "yo-yo" vicious circle of weight loss–weight gain) these diets also fail to address the many aesthetic and psychological aspects of weight loss and gain. (Specific diets are discussed later in this chapter, in the section "Why Even the Most Popular Diets Don't Work.")

DON'T COUNT CALORIES

A calorie is a unit of energy, and technically, the "large" calorie used in nutrition is one thousand of the "small" calories used in physics. In the body, calories are provided by the oxidation of food, a process which at bottom consists of the chemical reaction of carbon and hydrogen with oxygen to yield water and carbon dioxide. This oxidation supplies energy for movement, for warmth, and to drive other chemical reactions. The usual stand taken in diet books and in the popular press is that calories consumed must equal calories burned, otherwise a person puts on weight. A pound of body fat is the rough equivalent of 3,500 stored calories, and supposedly eating only 100 excess calories a day will cause weight gain of about a pound a month. Just reversing the process is said to take off the added pounds.

If this presentation were all that there is to the body's use of calories, then the companies that make a mint selling scales, calorie charts of common foods, and various prepared food items with their calories already counted should have succeeded long ago in putting an end to excess poundage in America. But there are still 70–80 million Americans who, despite considerable effort in some cases, have not been able to lose unwanted weight permanently. Why?

Part of the answer lies in the notion of metabolic individuality outlined previously. It is not just the food eaten, but the specific physiological attributes of the person eating the food that matters. Restricting calories may work wonders for the individual who gained weight solely because of a bout of inactivity and excess consumption, but whose metabolism has not been otherwise altered by the excess. This is the case with some—not all—women who gain weight during pregnancy and who afterward need a little help in losing it. Yet for those genetically disposed toward weight gain, for those who have gained too much weight and kept it long enough to alter their bodies regulatory mechanisms, and for those who for medical or other reasons have put on and kept on excess pounds, counting calories is usually a humiliating and futile exercise that does little or nothing to remove excess weight.

Energy requirements among individuals of the same age, sex, and apparent body composition can vary from person to person by as much as 100 percent. Even those with the same relative amount of lean tissue can exhibit unexplained variations of 25 percent![16] Moreover, the body is not passive in the face of a changing supply of calories. It constantly modifies its own energy expenditures in ways that make nonsense of simple calorie-in, calorie-out equations. How can it be the case that the woman not losing weight on 750 calories a day is not restricting her food intake sufficiently?

CARBOHYDRATES, FATS, AND ALCOHOL

As a rule, carbohydrates are the preferred source of energy. Of all foods, they burn the cleanest, producing only water and carbon dioxide as waste products. This means that carbohydrates place little burden upon the liver and kidneys. Carbohydrates likewise are the best source for the production of glycogen, a special sugar used and stored in the liver and in the muscles, and for the production of the blood sugar glucose that is needed by the brain. When carbohydrates are not available, the body breaks down protein—but not so readily fat—in order to supply the sugar necessary for brain function.

Fat supplies roughly twice the number of calories per gram (9 calories) as either carbohydrates or protein (4 calories each). Alcohol supplies 7 calories per gram. Although a certain amount of alcohol is routinely produced in the large intestine as a byproduct of the action of bacteria and yeast and is readily detoxified by the liver, and although small amounts of consumed alcohol actually improve health, in quantities beyond a couple of beers, or two or three glasses of wine, alcohol is toxic. Worse for the dieter, alcohol in any quantity inhibits the metabolism of fats, an action which itself involves the liver. Researchers reason that the liver must detoxify the alcohol before it can attend to the burning of fats, and this process slows fat metabolism by about a third.[17]

Fat may indeed have far more calories per gram than do other foods, but this does not mean that we can do without fats. There are a small number of polyunsaturated fats called essential fatty acids (EFAs) that the body cannot manufacture and that it cannot do without. Fats provide the basis for every hormone in the body and for essential components of all cell walls. Fats transport fat-soluble vitamins, such as A, D, and beta-carotene. Fats constitute the sheaths of all nerves. Finally, lipids, that is, fats, make up some 25 percent of the dry weight (the non-water weight) of brain tissue. As will be pointed out in this chapter, extremely low-fat diets, when followed for long periods of time, appear to damage or exhaust important systems in the body. Extremely low-fat diets (below 10 percent of all calories) have some recognized therapeutic uses, but they *are not* maintenance diets.

THE EFFECTS OF EXCESS CALORIES

Researchers in nutrition have shown that the results of the ingestion of a given number of calories depend upon many factors, the most important of which appear to be the following:

- The basal metabolic rate of the individual.
- The ratio of lean to fatty tissue of the individual.
- The degree and the duration of excess consumption.
- The amount of physical activity.
- The timing of food consumption, for example, when eaten during the day and when eaten in relation to physical activity.
- The source(s) of the calories; for example, whether protein, fat, and so on.
- The combination of sources of calories.
- Genetic factors, disease, or other unknown factors.

Weighing these various contributing factors properly can only be done on a case-by-case basis. However, there are some general rules that seldom are wrong.

First, it is possible for non-obese individuals with stable weights to modestly overconsume carbohydrates for periods of time without gaining weight. However, researchers generally agree that over long periods of time the consistent excess consumption of calories from carbohydrates (that is, consumption of calories well beyond energy requirements) will lead to fat storage. The degree of response depends upon each subject's metabolic identity.

Second, for most individuals on mixed diets—that is, diets combining protein, carbohydrates, and fats in the same diet—excessive amounts of fat are more likely to be stored as fat than are excessive amounts of carbohydrates. Reactions to mixed diets are greatly magnified, even distorted, when the carbohydrates are sugars or otherwise simple and refined in nature. Read on to find out why this is the case.

Third, an excess consumption of carbohydrates is known to increase the body's production of lipogenic (fat-storing) enzymes, such as lipoprotein lipase.[18] The overeating of carbohydrates for long periods of time increases the body's ability to store calories as fat. Sugars are especially implicated in this process.

Fructose, the sugar found in fruit, is particularly noted for stimulating lipogenesis (fat storage). Fructose, unlike glucose, does not require insulin for its movement from the blood into the cells, and for this reason it is listed as being very low on the glycemic index (20), an index that rates the degree of blood sugar elevation triggered by foods in comparison with that triggered by glucose (100 on the index). This has fooled many into thinking that fructose is a sugar that can be eaten in large amounts—and, indeed, we Americans do eat it in large amounts since we consume large amounts of fruit, especially as juices. Also fructose makes up about half the sugar in corn syrups and in this form is added to most American processed foods, even many meats! Almost all of the fructose eaten is converted into glucose (causing a delayed insulin peak), and in animal experiments fructose elevated triglyceride and insulin levels so consistently that researchers concluded that fructose was more damaging than other sugars, not less. Fructose also increases blood levels of uric acid, an effect that adds a burden to the kidneys and is involved in promoting gout.[19]

In general, the high level of sugar (sucrose, fructose, and so on) intake of the average American is implicated in chronic liver damage, fructose being perhaps the worst offender. Sugars cause significant increases in liver enzymes and, to repeat, the elevation of blood triglycerides. These findings suggest that the consumption of sugars can alter liver functions, perhaps permanently.[20]

Fourth, there is some evidence that the timing of meals is important. Calories eaten in the evening before bedtime are made available after the body has begun to slow down in preparation for sleep and, hence, are stored. Eating late in the evening also makes one inclined to skip breakfast, and not eating a meal early in the day signals the body to conserve energy while leading to excess food consumption at the first meal eaten. Eating breakfast both warms the body—that is, eating breakfast in itself encourages thermogenesis—and signals the body that it is free to expend energy without fear of famine. Breakfast eaters tend to snack less and to consume less total fat. Eating the same total number of calories, obese subjects who ate three full meals have been shown to lose more weight than those who ate only lunch and supper.[21] Eating calories from protein at breakfast, similarly, is more satiating than is the same caloric intake from carbohydrate.[22]

Fifth, getting regular exercise, in particular taking a short walk after meals, has many benefits. Moderate regular exercise (moderate here meaning merely twenty minutes, three times per week) has been shown to aid in preventing obesity, heart disease, colectoral cancer, and various psychological disorders.[23] Unfortunately, in the United States at the present time, only 37 percent of individuals at the most physically active stage of their lives, students in grades 9–12, regularly get moderate exercise; this is a decline from 62 percent in 1984.[24] The good news, however, is that modifying the diet with the addition of moderate exercise really does work![25]

Exercise helps to control blood sugar levels without bringing insulin into play. For this reason alone, exercise, especially a mild form immediately after meals, would be worthwhile. Insulin, which clears excess sugar from the blood, is one of the primary hormones involved in fat storage. Moderate exercise (aerobic only) also helps the body develop the ability to mobilize fat stores for energy. A brisk walk for thirty minutes twice a day raises the metabolic rate for a sustained period of time while helping to elevate the production of the enzymes that pull fat from storage. This process is called *lipolysis,* and it is commonly impaired in those who are overweight.[26] *Please note: The number of calories burned during the brief interval of exercise does not determine the value of the exercise.* The maintenance of lean tissues, the potentiation of insulin, and the raised basal metabolic rate all continue long after exercise is discontinued. Considerable research shows that moderate exercise can significantly increase insulin sensitivity and glucose tolerance, thus enabling the pancreas to produce less insulin.[27]

Dr. Grant Gwinup, Professor of Metabolism and Endocrinology at the University of California at Irvine, has rather neatly summed up the role of exercise in dieting as follows: "Exercising is far more effective than dieting in getting rid of excess weight. Individuals who diet without exercising lose mainly water and some muscle . . . When you're not eating enough food, when you're relying *only* on dieting to lose weight, your body fights back. It lowers your metabolic rate . . . However, if you exercise strenuously for 30 minutes or more daily, you will burn fat and keep muscle. You may not even have to cut down on food . . . Fat [also] is burned at a much faster rate."[28]

Sixth, increased consumption of dietary fiber, especially water-soluble fiber, is helpful for improving health and reducing excess weight. The bulk of the fiber itself gives a physical feeling of fullness, which helps to control how much is eaten at a given meal. Furthermore, the high bulk and water content associated with fiber tends to slow down the process of eating to a point at which feedback signals of satiety from the brain can influence hunger and appetite; similarly, intestinal hormones that reduce food intake can be released. Thus, appetite is reduced directly by the bulk of the fiber and indirectly through the delayed emptying of the stomach and the release of hormones signaling satiety.[29]

Vegetable sources of fiber, in particular, usually combine few calories with large amounts of vitamins and minerals. There is considerable evidence that these micronutrients, especially minerals such as chromium, are necessary for proper insulin and lipid control. Meanwhile, the bulking action of soluble fiber slows down the release of carbohydrates into the blood from the intestines. The moderate rise in blood sugar levels associated with complex carbohydrates, especially with vegetables and legumes, likewise moderates the release of insulin into the blood and avoids both the health dangers and the surges in appetite that characterize the body's responses to excessive insulin release.[30]

This last point brings up the issue of nutrition in general. A large amount of research suggests that the American diet, as a result of modern farming, storage techniques, and food processing, is routinely deficient in the minerals responsible for blood sugar and lipid control. Other research indicates that the modern consumption of refined oils and the consumption of oils derived from the sources that we find to be most plentiful and cheap interferes with the body's mechanisms for fat storage and energy production. (More on this in the next section—you may also wish to review the section on gamma-linolenic acid [GLA] in Chapter 2.)

Finally, genetics plays a powerful role in contributing to obesity. This point was mentioned above under the discussion of body types, but it should be pointed out that there are specific genes that now are implicated in both obesity and diabetes. Interestingly, these genes find expression under similar circumstances, that is, with a diet such as that followed in the United States, which is high in simple sugars, in fats, and in total calories, yet low in physical activity. They control the production of the enzyme G-6-PD (glucose-6-phosphate dehydrogenase). This enzyme, as its name suggests, is a sugar-storage enzyme that causes the conversion of sugar to fat for storage.[31]

THE USUAL CAUSE OF WEIGHT GAIN IN AMERICA

A study published in the *American Journal of Physiology* (September 1988) found that "even *small* amounts of mixed diet overfeeding will result mostly in fat storage, and lead to obesity if sustained for prolonged periods of time."[32] In a nutshell, this means that eating too many calories on a regimen that mixes fats and carbohydrates will almost certainly lead to fat storage. This should be amended to state *the consumption of fats in conjunction with simple carbohydrates in particular,* for it is simple carbohydrates that most markedly increase blood glucose levels and lead to derangements in insulin and lipid metabolism. If looked at from a historical perspective, this diet pattern describes exactly the nature of our changed eating habits as Americans have become heavier and more prone to sugar- and lipid-related disorders, such as heart disease and diabetes. Already in 1962 Dr. Margaret A. Ohlson presented the following picture of changes in the American diet, a picture largely maintained over the last forty years:

> Estimates of food available in retail channels per capita of population can be found in the reports of the U.S. Department of Commerce and, for recent years, the U.S. Department of Agriculture (for the period from 1889 to the present). Certain well marked trends can be identified. The consumer supplies of two basic sources of starch, i.e., cereals and potatoes, have decreased sharply. At the same time, the form of market cereals has changed from bread flour to highly processed bakery products and the prepared type of breakfast cereal. The per capita supply of refined sugar has increased from 50 pounds per person per year to about 100 pounds.[33]

The figure of per capita sugar consumption in the United States climbed until the 1980s with consumption peaking at about 120 pounds per year. Sugars of various derivations (for example, fructose) are now so commonly employed in hidden forms in almost all processed foods that keeping track of the actual figure has become very difficult. During this same period of time, total fat consumption remained largely stable with a small increase in polyunsaturated fats, which have steadily become a larger proportion of all fats consumed. Protein consumption by some estimates has actually declined slightly. Since an ever greater proportion of our food is processed, the amounts of various vitamins and minerals has declined absolutely. The addition of a few select vitamins and minerals after processing, and more recently the re-addition of fiber, is scarcely an adequate return. The immediate link between carbohydrates and vitamins and minerals that is found in all traditional sources of food has been broken by many modern techniques of storage, handling, and processing.[34]

The primary mechanism involved in weight gain on a mixed diet of fats and simple carbohydrates is that of insulin metabolism, and this data has been available since the 1930s. H. P. Himsworth early in that decade performed a number of dietary experiments in which subjects ate varying proportions of fat, protein, and carbohydrate for a week or so before being given the then standard glucose tolerance test for diabetes. This test elevates blood sugar levels by the administration orally of a controlled amount of the simple sugar dextrose, after which the amount of sugar in the blood is sampled at 30-, 60-, and 120-minute intervals. The evidence showed that the higher the percentage of all calories in the diet derived from fats in the interval before the test (usually a week), the higher the blood sugar levels after the administration of dextrose—that is, the higher the level of glucose tolerance and the greater the impairment of response to the release of insulin.[35]

These findings have sometimes been taken as an indictment of high-fat diets per se, but they actually prove exactly what they appear to prove, which is that sugars and other simple carbohydrates in the presence of fats cause an impaired insulin response. Fat metabolism uses different pathways than does carbohydrate metabolism, and the body cannot easily switch between the two, which is what the ingestion of simple carbohydrates—which now make up 40 percent of the American diet—demands. (The catabolic hormone glucagon, which mobilizes fat for energy and which also activates brown fat, or brown adipose tissue, suppresses the anabolic hormone insulin, and vice versa.) An impaired insulin response allows large amounts of sugar to enter the blood without being controlled, which results in the body's desperate release of far larger amounts of insulin. As more and more glucose enters the blood (too much is toxic), the body first turns this sugar into triglycerides (which make the blood thicker and "stickier") and then, via the now excessive amounts of insulin, these triglycerides are stored in fat cells. The presence of excess glucose in the blood itself interferes with the use of fat for energy and, through the action of the liver, again elevates the level of triglycerides and their storage as fat.[36] Fructose can be taken up in small amounts from the blood by the cells without the benefit of insulin. However, direct fructose metabolism is limited. Fructose can be fully eliminated from the blood only through the action of the liver, which converts fructose to glucose. The process of conversion merely delays the increase in the blood glucose levels, and it thereby delays the accompanying insulin spike. Significantly, a very large proportion of those who are overweight show signs of insulin resistance, and likewise, fully 80 percent of those who become diabetics as adults are over-weight.[37] This indicates that the routine experience of highly elevated levels of insulin release damages the ability to respond to this hormone, and insulin resistance and obesity are linked together in the vast prepon-derance of cases.

WHY AMERICANS ARE FATTER THAN THE FRENCH

The tendency toward a large percentage of the population carrying excess weight is a relatively recent phenomenon, and one much more characteristic of the United States than of Europe, as those who have traveled abroad can attest. For instance, the French in general show the diseases of excess and of age both less frequently and at a later point in life than their American counterparts; they are healthier and live longer despite smoking far more. Why? They eat four times as much butter as we do, more than twice as much cheese (commonly 60 or even 75 percent but-terfat), and about the same number of calories. Indeed, the French eat more than twice the animal fats and only two-thirds the supposedly healthful vegetable oils that Americans eat. *The French eat about half the whole milk and only one-eighteenth—that is right, only 5.6 percent!—the sugar consumed in this country.* (We Americans, like the British, are noto-rious for our love of sugar.[38]) The French even eat only about one-half the fruit we consume, and therefore about one-half the fructose from that source. (Since the French insist upon fresh foods, they avoid the fructose hidden in most processed foods.) On the other side of the ledger, the French consume more vegetables, more fish, more grains, more potatoes, and more of other complex carbohydrates.[39] They also do not snack between meals, a habit that has been shown in overweight individuals to increase the total daily consumption of calories. Interestingly, in the "graz-ing" versus "gorging" debate in diabetes research, the move from three meals to nine meals per day in a one-month study (as opposed to very short studies of one to a few days) demonstrated that the grazing approach did not improve glycemic control.[40]

According to the advice of the popular press, the American food industry, the American Medical Association, and so forth, the French are doing just about everything wrong. But according to the health statistics, they are doing something right, and that "something right" includes a diet with lots of fresh and whole, unprocessed foods, but rather low amounts of sugars of any sort. As mentioned, they eat one-eighteenth the amount of refined sugar found in the American diet and about half the sugar that we consume from fruit, and actually that figure may well understate how much more sugar we Americans actually consume. It is the American diet, one simultaneously high in both fats and simple carbohydrates, that bears a large degree of responsibility for American weight problems.

(Lest the reader think that the French are the only exception, it should be pointed out that the Swiss, who are second only to the Japanese among industrialized countries in life expectancy, eat even more in the way of cheeses, butter and cream, sausages, and so on, than do the French. No European group, however, appears to drink as much pasteurized and homogenized milk as Americans drink.)

If it is the American version of the mixed diet that is at fault for many of our health problems, including obesity, *then controlling the amount of fat in the diet is only one-half of any solution.* To be sure, the higher the percentage of calories in the diet that comes from fat, the greater the degree of sensitivity to the negative effects of simple carbohydrates. However, as long as simple carbohydrates remain an important part of the daily menu, even the relatively small amounts of fats necessary for nerve health, the workings of the immune system, the processing of fat-soluble vitamins, and so forth will continue to pose a critical challenge to weight control. This realization, moreover, is not new, but quite old. For instance, the ancient Indians of the Asian subcontinent began to use curry therapeutically because at least one of its chief ingredients, turmeric, controls excess reactions, that is, an elevated insulin response, to the "sweetness" of white rice. (see CHROMIUM, VANADYL SULFATE, AND OTHER INSULIN POTENTIATORS on page 23 in Chapter 2. Turmeric, along with cinnamon, cloves, bay leaves, and a number of other spices and herbs, potentiates the action of insulin.)

Overall, the dietary problems of Americans can be rectified to a large extent merely by returning to the consumption of primarily unprocessed foods, including oils, and of unprocessed complex carbohydrates in general; by the movement to the occasional use of low-glycemic-index grains (for example, more use of millet and barley, which in traditional medical systems are sometimes used to control diabetes, and less use of wheat and rice); by the reduction of the excessive consumption of fruit (especially as juice) and of any other sources of fructose; and by similar relatively minor dietary measures. To this regimen must be added a certain amount of moderate exercise to encourage the body to function properly. In those people whose systems have already been damaged, a few more steps may be necessary to correct faulty fat metabolism; for example, the addition of special essential fatty acids and other nutrients to daily foods.

HYPOTHYROIDISM, LIVER FUNCTION, AND BROWN FAT

Hypothyroidism refers to the insufficient activity of the thyroid gland. Symptoms of this condition include extreme fatigue, memory loss, depression, nervousness, allergies, sleep disturbances, menstrual disturbances, reduced sex drive, digestive disorders, and other problems. Inasmuch as the thyroid hormone plays a major role in controlling the expenditure of energy, in the liberation and metabolism of stored fats, and in determining the basal metabolic rate, the proper functioning of the thyroid is of considerable importance for the individual attempting to lose weight. Unfortunately, the refined diet characteristic of contemporary America tends to depress thyroid function.

The thyroid requires much more than just iodine to play its role in the body properly. Deficiencies of the vitamins A, B_2, C, and E, as well as of other nutrients, long have been known to reduce the activity of this gland, and many authorities doubt that the current recommended daily intakes of these vitamins are anywhere near adequate. Since low thyroid function is also correlated to excess blood lipid levels, it is clear that the various systems of the body are closely interrelated and that nutritional inadequacies affecting one system commonly spill over into and affect others. Those who are seriously overweight should have their basal body temperature and other indicators of thyroid function checked by a competent physician and make sure that they are consuming the nutrients important for thyroid function in adequate amounts.[41]

A second organ strongly linked to problems of fatigue and problems of sugar and fat metabolism is the liver. Liver dysfunction is found in a large percentage of overweight individuals,[42] and, as was pointed out previously, the consumption of refined sugars leads to liver damage.

Rather unfortunately, hypothyroidism can worsen the effects of liver dysfunction so that sufferers are more inclined to consume excess refined carbohydrates and gain weight.

It seems that in many cases of inadequate thyroid hormone secretion, the adrenal glands are influenced to reduce their own secretion of cortisol (hydrocortisone). Without the adrenal cortisol, the liver does not produce sufficient glycogen, its own special storage sugar also found in the muscles, and this deficiency leads indirectly to hypoglycemia, that is, to low or unstable blood sugar levels. Much the same situation arises with the excess release of insulin in response to the consumption of refined carbohydrates: the sufferer undergoes periods of extreme hunger despite the consumption of adequate numbers of calories.[43] (Also see "The Atkins Diet and Others Like It" on page 133.)

A special form of fatty or adipose tissue called brown fat makes up yet another aspect of the body's ability to regulate its energy consumption. Brown fat (brown adipose tissue, or BAT) is common in infants, but its quantity declines as we age. Found in the neck, along the spine and arteries, and around the most important internal organs, this fat is "brown" because of the high concentration of mitochondria, which are cellular components designed to generate energy. Brown fat is the single most important engine for the body's production of heat, that is, for thermogenesis, whereas the fat under the skin, which is white because of its lack of mitochondria, functions primarily as insulation and storage.

This difference is decisive—that is, brown fat's role in heat production versus normal fat's role in insulation and storage. In some people, brown fat may make up as much as 10 percent of all fat, while in others it may be only 1 or 2 percent. Inheritance is at least partly responsible for these varying amounts, and in animal studies it is clear that defective brown-fat function can cause obesity.[44] However, diet, the environment, and the degree of acquired heaviness all greatly influence matters. For instance, in response to cold and certain foods, the hypothalamus, the part of the brain that governs the sympathetic nervous system, releases the neurotransmitter noradrenaline (also called norepinephrine). Temperatures of about 72°F cause most fully clothed individuals to start to burn fat for heat. One of the drawbacks of obesity is its dampening of normal thermogenic responses. Not only does sustained obesity alter the hormonal balance that controls lipolysis, such as the balance between glucagon and insulin, but the insulating qualities of subcutaneous fat blocks the dissipation of body heat, and thus turns off the thermogenic functions of brown fat.[45]

Diet can promote the thermogenic action of brown fat by providing nutrient precursors to noradrenaline, such as phenylalanine, and by providing triggers and potentiators to the activity of noradrenaline, such as caffeine and ephedrine (from the herb ephedra or the Chinese herb ma huang). Diet also can interfere with thermogenesis. Excessive consumption of alcohol, saturated fats, caffeine, and *trans*-fatty acids such as are found in all margarines and most commercial vegetable oils; deficiencies of zinc, magnesium, and vitamin B_6; and cigarette smoking all interfere with the body's internal conversion of essential fatty acids into the fats necessary for thermogenesis and for general lipid metabolism.[46] (See again THERMOGENIC AIDS in Chapter 2.)

WHY EVEN THE MOST POPULAR DIETS DON'T WORK

Earlier we outlined the failings of radical and fad diets. Now that you have more information, it may prove useful to look more closely at some currently popular diet programs. This is intended to help the reader avoid making the mistake of blindly accepting the next "breakthrough" diet. There really are no "new" diets. All diets are variations of original themes discussed here. For convenience, the following brief review begins with the most austere diets and ends with the most luxurious.

Fasting

Undoubtedly one of the quickest ways to lose weight is to go on a complete fast. Under medical supervision, a fasting patient consuming only water might expect to lose about a pound a day, with men losing slightly more than women. This sounds impressive until it is realized that the weight being lost is up to 30 percent lean tissue, including tissue from the heart. Probably more disturbing for the individuals involved, in clinical trials of simple fasts, 90 percent or more of the patients regained all the weight they had lost within two years.

In any case, complete fasts require that one begin in relatively good health. Those with gout or other uric acid problems should avoid fasting. Also excluded are those with liver or kidney problems, those with circulatory diseases, those with anemia, and those with nervous disorders. Doctors overseeing fasts will not even allow their patients to take hot baths or showers because of the danger that the patients will faint, so the degree of disruption of normal bodily functions is clearly extreme.[47] Therefore, complete fasts should only be undertaken in the care of a physician under clinical conditions, and even if these conditions are met, total fasts are not recommended.

Fruit Diets and the Pritikin Diet

Quite a number of diet advocates base their diets on the consumption of fruit. One diet in this category is Judy Mazel's Beverly Hills Diet, and another is Harvey and Marilyn Diamond's Fit for Life diet. Their books, *The Beverly Hills Diet* and *Fit for Life* respectively, are almost identical in their basic claims, with the Diamonds paying attention primarily to the maintenance aspect of diet rather than any quick weight-loss program.

The Beverly Hills Diet brings together some quite reasonable points about food combining with some quite unrealistic expectations of what eating only fruit for two weeks will do for your weight. The advice about food combining is a reworking of the classic Hay System, a complete explanation of which can be found in Doris Grant and Jean Joice's book *Food Combining for Health* (Thorsons Publishers, 1987). That book should be consulted for a fuller presentation, but the basic points are these: proteins require an acid medium for digestion in the stomach, whereas starches require an alkaline medium in the small intestine, hence the two should not be eaten together. The claim is that eating a starch after consuming a protein actually results in the reduction of stomach-acid production despite the continued presence of the incompletely digested protein in the stomach. In the Hay System, fats in small amounts can be eaten with either proteins or carbohydrates, but in the Beverly Hills Diet, fats can be eaten only with carbohydrates.

The heart of the diet is a period of seven to ten days during which the dieter eats only fruit, and very little protein is added until the end of the third week. The third through the sixth weeks remain low in protein and low in cereal carbohydrates. Not surprisingly, people do lose weight on the diet, but then the caloric intake for the first two weeks is only about 500 calories a day.

There are several things wrong with fruit-based diets. First, protein deprivation during a pseudo-famine leads to large losses of both lean tissue and water from the body. The breakdown of lean tissue protein coupled with loss of water depletes the body of electrolytes, especially potassium, and this loss is aggravated by the diarrhea that usually accompanies the consumption of too much fruit. The result is muscular weakness, and, much more uncommonly, respiratory problems, renal (kidney) disorders, and cardiac irregularities.

Second, diets high in fruit are high in fructose. A variety of simple sugars are known to be damaging to the liver, and, as it has been pointed out, fructose in particular is noted for raising triglyceride levels and for disturbing fat metabolism in the body. Both the Beverly Hills Diet and that offered in *Fit for Life* fortunately separate fruit consumption from the consumption of other foods—*Fit for Life* is even more insistent on this point. Hence, these diets at least do not mix simple carbohydrates and fats. But such a high consumption of fruit is not healthful and merely panders to the American taste for things sweet.

The Diamonds and Judy Mazel live in a warm climate (Southern California) and recommend diets suitable only for an area where, or for seasons during which, the body's main problem is getting rid of excess heat. Those living elsewhere in harsher climates are unlikely to find this fruit diet so attractive. Likewise, take a close look at the skin of anyone who has eaten massive amounts of fruit for a long time—their skin most likely will display the dryness, wrinkles, and other signs of aging that characterize the cross-linkage of sugars and proteins that occur after exposure to sun on a diet high in sugars.

Fruit diets are unlikely to be successful for any length of time. The quick weight loss that accompanies fruit diets will cause the loss of valuable lean tissue and thus initiate the "yo-yo" effect unless the dieter remains on a radical diet plan. The maintenance diets proposed by Judy Mazel and the Diamonds are themselves unhealthy, and probably not endurable for anyone living in a cold climate. There is a final flaw in these diets, and that is the radical reduction in the consumption of fats and oils. This point is best discussed in the context of the Pritikin Diet.

The famous Pritikin Diet was established many years ago by Nathan Pritikin. It cuts salt and caffeine, pares sugars and other simple carbohydrates to 100 grams per day, cuts meat consumption to one-quarter of a pound per day, advocates the consumption of carbohydrates, and, most important, insists that fats and oils should constitute at best 10 percent of daily calories, but preferably only 5 percent. This last, lower figure is difficult to achieve inasmuch as even most whole grains contain a greater percentage than this of their calories as fats.

There is little doubt that, at least in its early phases, going on the Pritikin Diet has some strong therapeutic benefits for many people. Blood cholesterol levels tend to come down rapidly, as much as 50 percent of type 2 (adult-onset) diabetes patients become free of dependence on injected insulin, hypertension is reduced in as little as two weeks, and weight is usually normalized. As a short-term therapeutic diet, it is a success.

Nevertheless, there has proved to be a very large downside to long-term adherence to the Pritikin program. The diet is extraordinarily restrictive and requires considerable time in preparation. It promotes an overdependence upon grains, and this exaggerates problems of gluten intolerance. Gluten is a protein found in many grains, and even in non-sensitive individuals its excessive consumption can cause bloating and intestinal gas, diarrhea, fatigue, and mental instability. The insoluble-fiber content of many of these grains proves to be too much for most people, and at the levels found in the Pritikin Diet the total fiber content actually drains minerals from the body. Yeast-related problems appear in a significant number of those on the Pritikin Diet. Finally, these problems are not helped by the fact that those on this diet have tended to consume too much fruit and to use too much apple juice and other fruit juice concentrates for sweetening, thus elevating triglyceride levels.

Most of the foregoing criticisms of the Pritikin Diet, it should be pointed out, are those of a former director of nutrition at the main Pritikin Longevity Center in Santa Monica, California.[48] Moreover, the diet is at least marginally deficient in the fats needed to carry fat-soluble vitamins to nourish the brain and nerves and to feed the immune system. Indeed, the ingestion of less than 5 percent of daily calories as fat is associated with cancer, just as is consumption of fats in excess.[49] At its recommended 7 percent level of calories from fats, the Pritikin Diet is marginal in terms of the fat consumption required for long-term health. (See THE CHOLESTEROL CONTROVERSY on page 141 in Chapter 6.)

The moral of this story, then, is all things in moderation. Keep in mind that there are many variations on the theme of radical reduction in calories and of the use of some special component(s) in the diet. So-called zen macrobiotic diets (brown rice diets), for instance, fall into this category, and a number of people have died on such diets from malnutrition. Although one is unlikely to perish from simple malnutrition on the Pritikin Diet, several studies, both in the United States and in Europe, of people on similar extremely low-fat diets have shown disturbing increases in mortality rates from accidents, acts of violence, and suicides. The most likely explanation is damage to the central and peripheral nervous systems and/or inadequate production of brain chemicals due to inadequate fats in the diet.

Liquid Diets and Diet Powders

There are now so many liquid diets and diet powders that it is impossible to describe more than a small number. Most of these diets are versions of high-protein, low-fat, low-carbohydrate diets. Many are neither particularly good nor particularly bad in and of themselves, just expensive. The first point to consider is that such diets become unsafe if used to exclude too many calories. Consuming fewer than 800 calories a day without adequate supervision can lead to severe illness or even death by starvation. This may seem odd to those attempting to lose weight, but it actually can happen and must not be discounted.

Liquid protein diets containing neither fats nor carbohydrates, once a rage, are now thankfully much rarer, for they posed serious health hazards.[50] Protein diets of these sorts do little good unless the protein is of high quality and adequate vitamins and minerals are included. This seldom was or is the case. Without small amounts of carbohydrates, low-calorie, high-protein diets lead to large fluid losses and corresponding losses of electrolytes; they also lead to fatigue.[51] Moreover, the issue of fats comes up with any diet that increases protein and radically restricts oils and fats. Too much protein unbalanced by fat can lead to a special form of starvation. In pioneer days this was called "rabbit fever" after the fact that a diet made up exclusively of rabbits and other lean wild game caused severe illness. Indeed, some of the current arguments among university anthropologists over whether humans evolved as "hunters" or as "scavengers" revolve around the issue of which of these provided enough fat for a sustainable diet.[52]

Now on the market are various diet powders that are usually added to water and used in place of one or more meals. As with the liquid protein diets, the quality of the protein and the addition of other ingredients are of utmost importance. Nutrients beyond the usual vitamins and minerals are sometimes included (you can check these ingredients against the information on each in Chapter 2). An insignificant amount of fiber is sometimes added. More commonly, various sweeteners are added to make the drinks palatable. Fructose is a favorite sweetener since it is dubiously thought not to cause fat storage since, as discussed earlier, its ingestion is not immediately linked to the release of insulin but rather causes a delayed blood-sugar peak after conversion to glucose by the liver.

The best of these diet powders offer convenience, but few significantly influence the body to burn fat rather than protein or otherwise grossly affect energy metabolism. With their small amounts of fiber, if used for more than one meal a day, such diets are damaging for the simple reason that they interfere with the proper elimination of toxins through the bowels. Likewise, very-low-calorie, high-protein diets do little to train the dieter for life after the diet. Finally, if a given diet moves too close to dependence upon protein for calories, it then has all the drawbacks of the original and now discredited high-protein diets. That is, pure protein diets put stress on the liver and the kidneys, increase uric acid in the blood, and thus encourage gout; they ultimately promote the loss of lean tissue if they are too low in calories or are continued for too long a period of time.

The only very-low-calorie, high-protein products that appear to have real effects are those used medically. One such product popularized a decade ago by Dr. Connelly makes use of nutritional signals to direct energy utilization, a process Connelly terms "partitioning." Such agents "increase oxygen consumption and metabolic carbon dioxide production at the expense of fat storage independent of energy intake."[53] Partitioning agents were new in 1990, but they are old hat in 2003. (For more on partitioning agents, see the following sections in Chapter 2: CONJUGATED LINOLEIC ACID (CLA) on page 30, GAMMA-LINOLENIC ACID (GLA), FLAX, AND THE OMEGA-3 ESSENTIAL FATTY ACIDS on page 48, THERMOGENIC AIDS on page 73, and THYROID NUTRIENTS AND ACTIVATORS on page 80.)

The Atkins Diet and Others Like It

High-fat diets were used at the turn of the century to treat type 1 diabetes, the form that begins in childhood with the destruction of the insulin-producing cells of the pancreas. Since the body can and will produce its own blood sugar from protein in order to feed the brain, there is always some role for insulin in the body regardless of the diet followed. Needless to say, people with juvenile diabetes invariably died young until the discovery of insulin, and no diet could prevent this.

In adult-onset or type 2 diabetes, which typically begins fairly late in life, diet and exercise often can completely control the problem in those who are already overweight. This evidence, in addition to other clues, has led a number of researchers to suspect that excess weight gain is related to insulin production either directly or indirectly. Dr. Robert C. Atkins was one of the first to popularize the notion of dieting by bypassing the insulin mechanism through eliminating most carbohydrates from the diet while continuing to consume both proteins and fats. The Atkins Diet is both high in protein *and* high in fat.

As already discussed, high-protein, low-fat, very-low-carbohydrate diets have been common for some time, but not with the particular justification that they bypass the insulin mechanism. Generally the justifications have had to do with energy production, or rather the lack of it, on these diets. In the Stillman Diet, for instance, it was argued that protein molecules are so large that they use up extra energy as a food for the body. This diet calls for the drinking of at least eight glasses of water a day, which truly is necessary to remove the waste products of excess protein consumption and from the oxidation of the body's own fats. Very similar is the famous Scarsdale Diet, designed to be used for only two weeks at a time. Both diets strictly limit carbohydrates and, somewhat less strictly, fats. Both reduce weight in the short term, but with the downside that such large amounts of protein are extremely hard on the body, as already explained.

In contrast to these, the Atkins Diet allows for unlimited amounts of both proteins and fats, but for restricted amounts of carbohydrates according to the theory that a faulty insulin mechanism is the cause of excess weight. Dr. Atkins also includes a long list of supplements with his diets. At least two of his books specifically take aim at his many critics. (See *Dr. Atkins' Health Revolution*, 1989, and *Dr. Atkins' New Diet Revolution*, 1992.) These works provide a great deal of useful information about insulin metabolism, and they provide even more useful medical references. More recently, Dr. Atkins has moved to topics that include aging and alternatives to pharmaceutical drugs. (See, for example, *Dr. Atkins' Age-Defying Diet Revolution*, 2000, and *Dr. Atkins' Vita-Nutrient Solution*, 1998.) The string of published works from this prolific iconoclast has now come to an end. Dr. Atkins died in early 2003 from injuries sustained in a fall on an icy sidewalk.

There is no doubt that for weight loss, the Atkins Diet works. Fat stores are used for energy, and hunger disappears as the body begins to use ketones, which are fatty acids produced by the liver from fat, as its primary energy source. Those who are overweight often have difficulty mobilizing fats for energy in exercise or for other reasons, so the diet works by forcing the body to metabolize lipids via a different metabolic pathway. As with followers of the Pritikin Diet, those who stick to the Atkins Diet routinely discover that insulin production declines, blood pressure declines, and mood swings may disappear. A more limited form of this ketone-based diet is presented by Dr. Calvin Ezrin in *The Endocrine Control Diet* (1990).

The usual criticisms of the Atkins Diet include warnings of the potential for kidney damage and cardiovascular degeneration. Even the proponent of quite a similar diet program, Dr. Ezrin himself, faults Atkins's allowance for unlimited fat consumption on the grounds that this may lead to ketosis, which causes dehydration, and to damaging changes in blood chemistry as the blood becomes more acidic and calcium is depleted. However, this charge is a bit misplaced since the Atkins Diet does *not* restrict *all* carbohydrates. The Atkins Diet, in essence, depends upon the fact that the same *catabolic* enzymes are brought into play whether fat comes from the diet or from the body's own stores, and these enzymes can be derailed by the introduction of the *anabolic* enzyme insulin, which must be used to clear excess sugar from the blood. The Atkins Diet allows for as much as 60 grams of carbohydrate a day—about one-seventh of a pound daily—divided among all three meals. This amount of carbohydrate is roughly the same as that allowed on the best of the very-low-calorie, high-protein diets on the market.

Many in the medical profession simply assert that Atkins is wrong in his diet prescription because he flies in the face of current attitudes toward fat consumption. Inasmuch as Atkins has been able to provide quite considerable clinical data showing that his diet does not increase blood lipid levels, but the reverse, the issue is not simple. Indeed, a number of top bodybuilders in the World Bodybuilding Federation adopted a diet similar to the one Atkins uses (roughly 40 percent of calories from protein and 60 percent from fat) in order to cut body fat and build muscle! These individuals were all undertaking extremely hard physical labor, so the diet itself cannot be a source of fatigue, but must in fact supply considerable energy.[54] Therefore, the evidence is that the diet may have a valuable therapeutic role.

As of 2003, Atkins has received considerable vindication at the expense of his critics, even in articles in major medical journals, for instance in *The New England Journal of Medicine* (348[21]; [22 May 2003]:

2074–81, 2082–90). On July 7, 2002, *The New York Times* ran a very long article by Gary Taubes entitled, "What If It's All Been a Big Fat Lie?" Taubes, in very little space, points out that the world has been turned upside down. He begins by noting that the American Medical Association has attacked the Atkins Diet as a "bizarre regimen" and that Atkins had been forced to defend his diet in person at Congressional hearings. Despite such official condemnation, according to Taubes, Atkins and others touting similar messages have established themselves as one pole in the diet debate.

> . . . America has become weirdly polarized on the subject of weight. On the one hand, we've been told with almost religious certainty by everyone from the surgeon general on down, and we have come to believe with almost religious certainty, that obesity is caused by the excessive consumption of fat, and that if we eat less fat we will lose weight and live longer. On the other, we have the ever-resilient message of Atkins and decades' worth of best-selling diet books, including "The Zone," "Sugar Busters" and "Protein Power" to name a few. All push some variation of what scientists would call the alternative hypothesis: it's not the fat that makes us fat, but the carbohydrates, and if we eat less carbohydrates we will lose weight and live longer.

Taubes goes on to observe that the alternative explanation for obesity proposed by Atkins and others identifies as the culprit the same low-fat diet that has been prescribed for decades as the source of good health by medical authorities. Promoted endlessly at taxpayer expense, the low-fat-diet orthodoxy until about five years ago reigned virtually unchallenged in scientific circles. Taubes, as have other commentators, draws attention to the odd fact that even to propose testing the validity of the alternative hypothesis, that is, that it is carbohydrates rather than fats that lead to obesity, risked a scientist's reputation. A parallel situation with regard to the debate over hormone replacement therapy (HRT) for women is examined in the next chapter. That debate has now concluded—after decades of medical support as being self-evidently therapeutic, HRT is now admitted to be medically harmful in a significant percentage of cases. As with HRT, it has been a case of catch-22 for proponents of the alternative diet explanation: they were routinely accused of having no scientific data to back up their claims, yet no reputable scientist would risk his or her reputation to perform the trials needed to test the hypothesis that carbohydrates play a leading role in causing weight gain.

In the section "Why Americans Are Fatter Than the French" on page 124, it was argued that the evidence that eating fat makes one fat is opposed by numerous counterexamples from around the world. A few researchers, such as Loren Cordain at Colorado State University, long have argued against basing the official dietary recommendations on the proposition that carbohydrates are good and fats are bad. However, the carbohydrate foundation of the official Food Pyramid was not truly shaken until researchers such as Walter Willet at the Harvard School of Public Health weighed in on the controversy. These new academic heretics note that the current obesity epidemic began in the early 1980s and coincides with the triumph of the all-fat-is-bad school of thought, a point already touched on in 1993 in the first edition of *Anti-Fat Nutrients*. In both clinical trials and in real life, low-fat diets have failed. For two or more decades, the amount of fat in the American diet has been declining, as have serum cholesterol and rates of smoking. Oddly, these changes have not been matched by similar reductions in the incidence rate of heart disease. Taubes in his *New York Times* article quotes Willett as observing that this seeming paradox is "very disconcerting. It suggests that something else bad is happening."

Despite this reversal of fortune, it is not likely that the Atkins Diet is advisable as a maintenance diet. Excess protein is damaging to the kidneys and it tends to draw calcium out of the bones if not consumed in conjunction with adequate vegetables.[55] Eskimos eating their native diet of raw meat and blubber may be vigorous in youth and middle age, but they seldom live much past the age of sixty, and the women begin to show signs of calcium loss (osteoporosis) by the age of thirty. Likewise, modern Greenlanders living on a similar diet are vigorous, yet live short lives. But cooking meat actually turns it into a far greater burden on our immune systems during digestion than does eating it raw. Since it is to be doubted that Atkins expected, or anyone else expects, modern Americans to live primarily on raw meat, it is hard to believe that the continuous consumption of so much protein over the long term can be a good thing. Moreover, overshadowing its role in our metabolism proper, a large amount of dietary fat is often quite dangerous because of what the bacteria do to it in the intestines and because of the dangers of peroxidation within our tissues. This drawback should be considered when evaluating any diet.[56]

In conclusion, the Atkins Diet may actually be a good short-term diet for losing weight and for stabilizing insulin levels. As proof of the dangers of the usual American mixed diet of fats and simple carbohydrates, and as an indication of what can be accomplished by abandoning such a diet, it is also useful. Indeed, it is difficult not to conclude that the diet is preferable to the usual mixed diet based upon equal parts of protein, fats, and simple carbohydrates; for example, the burger, white bun, sweet "special" sauce, and fries served at fast-food restaurants. However, again it must be stressed that this does not mean that the Atkins Diet is the best maintenance diet over the long haul. Both the Atkins Diet and the Pritikin Diet, albeit from opposite extremes, primarily offer therapeutic intervention into the body's hormonal mechanism for controlling sugar and lipid metabolism. (Have another look at Chapter 4 for an example of a more realistic maintenance diet.)

The Barry Sears Diet

A good maintenance diet should contain some fat, and it is very unlikely that the 10 to 20 percent figure commonly suggested by dieting gurus is the correct one. Research has shown that reduced-calorie diets, whether high in carbohydrates or high in fat—yes, fat!—lead to very similar levels of weight loss. The same point can be made regarding longevity diets. Reducing the fat content in the diet has *not* proven to be the important variable; only reducing total calories has made a difference in longevity. Even the standard claim that eating fat leads to a higher intake of calories seems dubious. When normal-weight healthy men were tested under clinical conditions, it was found that a high-fat diet did *not* increase calorie intake when compared with low- and medium-fat diets, as long as the caloric density of the foods remained similar. (Protein intake was 12 percent of calories.) This means that fats eaten as part of a diet containing a reasonable amount of fiber do not increase the intake of calories—as opposed to fats eaten in calorie-dense forms, such as pastries, fast foods, or bonbons.

Indeed, if the fat content of the diet is too low, this may actually have a negative impact upon the ultimate calorie-burning result of exercise. Individuals who metabolize fat preferentially for energy (those who are high-fat oxidizers) benefit more from exercise as a means of losing or maintaining weight than those who burn primarily carbohydrates. The reason for this is simple: high-fat oxidizers spare glycogen stores (the limited carbohydrates stored in our bodies) as they burn fat for fuel; after the exercise is over, the high-fat oxidizers are not driven to eat excessively to restore the glycogen in the body. Low-fat oxidizers, however, must eat to replenish this necessary balance of body carbohydrate. Since the *relative* ability of the overweight to access their own fat stores is usually less (you wear it because you don't burn it), this suggests that a maintenance diet should contain a moderate amount of fat. A problem for dieters is that, although they have considerable fat of their own to burn for fuel, their glycogen stores are already only 50 percent or even as low as 20 percent of what these should be. Thus, dieters often find themselves forced to eat after exercise even though they may be burning fat fuel.

This brings us to Barry Sears and *The Zone*. Sears advocates a diet that consists of 30 percent protein, 30 percent fat, and 40 percent carbohydrate divided into small meals throughout the day. The aim of the diet is to maintain very even levels of insulin and blood sugar. Sears also claims that the high protein content of his diet releases the hormone glucagon, which opposes many of the actions of insulin. A few readers may notice that Sears has taken some points made originally by Heller and Heller in *The Carbohydrate Addict's Diet* and pushed these very far.

The chief argument is that about 25 percent of Americans naturally are resistant to the effects of insulin and therefore require more and more of it to maintain the balance of sugar in the blood if they eat carbohydrates. High insulin levels prevent fat from being burned and force it into storage. Those who are insulin resistant, therefore, are likely to have problems with a diet high in carbohydrates. For instance, if you find that eating a normal breakfast containing plenty of carbohydrates actually makes you tired and hungry, but that eating nothing or eating mainly protein for breakfast keeps you wide awake, then you may be insulin resistant. Sears maintains that an additional 50 percent of the population may develop insulin resistance if they follow a diet high in carbohydrates, such as that prescribed by most medical authorities.

In terms of active weight loss, these issues have already been discussed. Therapeutic diets usually restrict *either* carbohydrates *or* fats. If fats are restricted, then the diet will tend toward an increased protein content. Most dieters will find that in the early stages, this high intake of protein will reactivate the thyroid and make life easier. There is plenty of clinical evidence to the effect that high-protein snacks reduce calorie intake more than do snacks of carbohydrate, fat, or alcohol for overweight individuals accustomed to the usual American mixed diet. And increasing protein intake from 12 to 25 percent of calories clinically has been demonstrated to increase both weight loss (by 75 percent) and fat loss (by 57 percent).

However, there is nothing magical about the 30/30/40 ratio proposed by Barry Sears. One wag once pointed out to the authors that the great innovation of Barry Sears was to remind us that vegetables are the most healthful sources of carbohydrates. As indicated previously, if sugars and refined carbohydrates are avoided, and if half or more of each meal's plate is covered with lightly cooked vegetables (that is, there is a goodly quantity of fiber, mineral, and antioxidants in the diet), then the rest of the diet will tend to take care of itself. It is the fiber and the mineral contents of the diet that commonly separate the thin from the fat. As noted in the section on fiber in Chapter 2, overweight individuals typically eat far less fiber than do thin individuals. Likewise, research has shown that even a 32 percent sugar diet, which reliably makes test animals fat, does not do so when the diet is enriched with minerals. Finally, individuals eating the Mediterranean diet, which typically includes 35 to 40 percent fats, only 10 percent protein, and 50 to 55 percent carbohydrates, not only have the best record of longevity in the world, but also have a diet that tastes great! Enough said.[57]

CHAPTER 6

The Cholesterol Controversy

2004 PREFACE

In any book that takes on the subject of fat and related issues, it is necessary to say some words about cholesterol—the longtime, nearly mythological nemesis of many a dieter.

It is sometimes remarked that medical "truths" often are reversed every thirty or forty years. In mid-2002, this observation was borne out with a vengeance in the case of hormone replacement therapy (HRT). Long promoted as being heart protective and having a track record going back to roughly 1975, HRT was discovered to actually increase the rate of heart attack—and several other causes of death—in women.[1] Even the benefits against fracture risks appear to have been greatly overstated.[2] Interestingly, some epidemiologists never bought into the promises of HRT.[3] More curious still is the fact that the increased rates of heart disease in women on HRT resulted despite the fact that several cardiovascular disease "markers" or "risk factors," such as cholesterol levels, were significantly decreased.

A similar reversal is slowly taking shape in the area of research concerned with cardiovascular disease, markers of blood lipids, and cholesterol-lowering drugs. The theory that dietary cholesterol intake is the primary contributor to cardiovascular disease has not been well supported by dietary intervention trials. Similarly, prior to the advent of the statin drugs, which work by non-cholesterol mechanisms, decades of use of pharmaceuticals that strikingly lower serum lipids has not resulted in reductions in the death rate from heart disease. The authors of this book have updated this chapter to take into account recent studies and events, and to make the analysis current as of late 2003. However, most of the materials and conclusions below are the same ones found in the first edition of *Anti-Fat Nutrients* published in the spring of 1993. This means that sufficient evidence was present a decade ago to conclude that the role of cholesterol in cardiovascular disease, and certainly that of the dietary intake of cholesterol, was, at best, overstated and, at worst, completely wrong-headed. For a good overview of the direction the controversy has taken of late, one should read the July 7, 2002, *New York Times* article by Gary Taubes entitled "What if It's All Been a Big Fat Lie?" As in the case of HRT, a disproportionately large percentage of epidemiologists have been skeptical of the claims of the cholesterol theory of heart disease.[4] Those individuals seriously interested in this topic should read Uffe Ravnskov, *The Cholesterol Myths* (NewTrends Publishing, 2000).

To be sure, Ravnskov does not consider at length the multitude of new markers and cholesterol subclasses presently being researched. Many studies performed over the last decade demonstrate that the sizes of the various subclasses of HDL and LDL cholesterol are more predictive of heart disease risk than are levels of LDL, HDL, and total cholesterol. Larger particles of LDL are less atherogenic (damaging to the walls of the arteries) than are smaller particles, larger particles of HDL are more effective at carrying LDL back to the liver for disposal than are smaller HDL particles, and so on. Also, there are other blood lipids and markers that have been shown to be risk indicators of heart attack and heart disease: lipoprotein(a), homocysteine, intermediate-density lipoproteins, apolipoprotein B, apolipoprotein E4, and so forth. However, the standard lipid panel does not provide this information, and moreover, the entire cholesterol theory was put forward and defended for forty years without such information. The cholesterol theory, if evaluated by way of its original evidence and argument, is clearly unsubstantiated, and the new data, in turn, may end up fitting other explanatory paradigms much better than they do the cholesterol theory.

Likewise, the recommendations based upon the cholesterol theory, such as radically reduced-fat diets, either have failed when put to the test or yielded such trivial results that significance has been achieved only by studying massive numbers of individuals. A recent review of low-fat diets found that a reduction in dietary fat was associated with reduced cardiovascular morbidity, but not reduced total mortality. The finding that cardiovascular deaths were reduced by 9 percent, and cardiovascular events by 16 percent—the positive finding—fell when the

Oslo Diet-Heart Trial, which examined the effects of fish oil, was excluded. With this exclusion, cardiovascular deaths were reduced by 6 percent, cardiovascular events by 14 percent, but overall death rates actually increased 2 percent. Fish oil, of course, contains omega-3 fatty acids.[5] The best that can be said after forty years regarding the simple reduction of fat in the diet is, as the authors of the Cochrane Review, a major medical review, recently concluded, "findings are suggestive of a small but potentially important reduction in cardiovascular risk in trials longer than two years."[6] This on diets in which the intervention obviously would have led to changes in more than just fat consumption, hence it is likely that the positive outcomes, such as they were, reflected factors other than just reductions in fat intake. (For those readers who are wondering how an assessment of low-fat diets could be positive even though life expectancy was not improved, we have no answer.) The critical assessments of the same decades of dietary intervention by a research group associated with Walter Willet at Harvard points out that, "metabolic studies have long established that the type of fat, but not total amount of fat, predicts serum cholesterol levels."[7] Readers who want a balanced view of what diets can and cannot do from an authority on eating habits from around the world should read Walter C. Willett's book *Eat, Drink, and Be Healthy* (Simon & Schuster Source, 2001). Willett's "food pyramid" looks nothing like the one presently being pushed by the FDA and the American Heart Association.

Public health authorities loudly trumpet the reduction in coronary heart disease over the last thirty years as evidence of the success in steadily reducing the level of fat in the American diet over the same period. Such claims pale a bit when placed against the backdrop of steadily rising rates of obesity, diabetes, hypertension, data from 1987–1994 showing stable or increasing rates of heart attack, and so on. What is really going on? It is actually quite simple: medical intervention after the attack, and not prevention, is at work in these claims to success. This fact was pointed out in the earlier editions of *Anti-Fat Nutrients,* and it has been borne out, yet again, by more recent reevaluations of data from the late 1980s and early 1990s. When scientists at the School of Public Health at the University of North Carolina, Chapel Hill, looked at the relationship between new cases of heart attack and the rate of death from heart disease, they found the former was actually increasing during the period of their study, whereas the latter was going down.

*From 1987–1994, we observed a stable or slightly increasing incidence of
hospitalization for myocardial infarction. Nevertheless, there were significant annual decreases in mortality from CHD (coronary heart disease). The decline in mortality in the four communities we studied may
be due largely to improvements in the treatment and secondary prevention of myocardial infarction.[8]*

Statistical analyses based on data running through the end of the
1990s indicate that declines in in-hospital CHD mortality during that
decade were nearly three times greater than declines in out-of-hospital
mortality.[9] Such statistics indicate that at least three-quarters of the modern reduction in deaths from coronary heart disease has come from hospital interventions. All other factors combined, such as the much-touted
changes in dietary-fat intake and the widespread prescription of choles-
terol-reducing medications and a host of other drugs, likely accounts for
no more than 25 percent of the improvement.

No other author comes anywhere close to providing the thoroughness
exhibited by Dr. Ravnskov's dissection of the cholesterol theory of heart
disease. He and other critics also take on the new treatments using the
statin class of drugs. These critics argue that the statins do not work by
influencing cholesterol levels, but rather by reducing inflammation in
the artery wall and by directly inhibiting the proliferation of the smooth
muscle of the arterial endothelium. Indeed, the impact of these drugs
upon the synthesis of cholesterol likely is undesirable because drugs that
inhibit this synthesis in the manner of the statins also inhibit the production of coenzyme Q_{10}, hence leading to increases in deaths from car-
diomyopathy, and so on, and to declines in health in other areas, such as
cognitive functioning. In light of the emerging research linking cardiovascular diseases ever more closely to inflammatory processes and ever
more distantly to cholesterol as such, the conclusions found in the earlier
editions of *Anti-Fat Nutrients* begin to appear prescient.

❦

cholesterol n. a fatlike material . . . present in the blood and most
tissues, especially nervous tissue. Cholesterol and its esters are
important constituents of all cell membranes and are precursors
of many steroid hormones and bile salts. Western dietary intake
is approximately 500–800 mg/day. Cholesterol is synthesized in

the body from acetate, mainly in the liver, and blood concentration is normally 150–250 mg/100 ml. . . . Elevated blood concentration is often associated with atheroma (arteriosclerosis accompanied by pronounced degenerative changes), of which cholesterol is a major component. Cholesterol is also a constituent of gallstones.[10]

Of all possible health risks, the two with which Americans are most familiar are smoking and cholesterol. The reason that most of us are familiar with cholesterol, aside from its constant presence in the media, is that coronary heart disease remains the leading cause of death in the United States. Almost everyone at one point or another has learned that elevated blood levels of cholesterol may be hazardous to health. Out of a concern for controlling cholesterol levels through dietary means, whole new categories of foods are now being created, such as inassimilable artificial fats for use in mayonnaise, in ice cream, and so forth. Similarly, vegetable oils now are used in place of animal fats by major fast-food chains for frying purposes, and the list goes on.

The usual rendition of the health hazards of cholesterol runs as follows: Dietary fats, especially animal and other saturated fats, are readily absorbed by the body and/or cause the liver to produce fats known as low-density lipoproteins (LDLs), which damage the walls of the major arteries and other blood vessels. Cholesterol then collects at these damaged sites and narrows the vessels until blood cannot pass. In classic coronary artery disease, vessels that supply blood to the heart are blocked, and the heart is starved for nutrients and oxygen. Alternatively, as in the case of many strokes, cholesterol narrows the blood vessels that feed the brain. Eating a diet low in saturated fats and cholesterol lowers the risk of cardiovascular and related diseases.

The problem with this picture is that it does not appear to be entirely true! There are many things that can be done to reduce the risks of heart disease and strokes, but removing fats from the diet is a fairly minor factor. Before delving into what can be done to lower our risks, a brief look at the present state of research on cholesterol and heart disease is in order.

In 1992 one of the most prestigious of all journals devoted to the study of heart and circulatory diseases, *Circulation,* published an article entitled "Health Policy on Blood Cholesterol: Time to Change Directions." The authors of this article evaluated the best studies on lowering cholesterol through dietary and drug intervention that we have on record and came to these conclusions:

- In both men and women, low blood cholesterol readings are associated with elevated mortality rates from non-cardiovascular diseases. Readings below 160 in men may actually be associated with slight increases in cardiovascular disease, as are readings above 200.

- In women, high blood cholesterol levels have no association with deaths from cardiovascular disease.

- In the major long-term intervention studies, whether these used dietary or drug means for lowering serum cholesterol levels, reduced mortality rates from cardiovascular causes were offset by increased mortality rates from non-cardiovascular causes in those populations not already characterized by heart disease.[11]

It should be pointed out that other similar findings have received considerable airing on the research side of the medical community. For instance, at the November 14, 1991, annual meeting of the American Medical Association, Dr. Peter Wilson reported that the rates of heart attack and of angina have not been lowered over the past decade. Death rates have declined almost entirely because of improved techniques of intervention and treatment, not because of a lowered incidence of attack.[12] This is true despite the steady decline of saturated fats and cholesterol as components of the American diet.

Several recent books and booklets have covered in great depth the failure of the cholesterol hypothesis to account for most heart disease. Among these are *Heart Myths* by Bruce D. Charash, M.D. (Viking, 1991), *Heart Failure* by Thomas J. Moore (Touchstone/Simon and Schuster, 1990), and "The Facts and Myths about Coronary Heart Disease" by the American Council on Science and Health (September 1989).

The most troubling aspect of the recent turnabout in attitudes toward cholesterol, leaving aside the realization that the American public has remained almost in the dark, is that none of the doubts about the cholesterol hypothesis are new. The same report thirty years ago that led the U.S. Surgeon General to require that all cigarette packages bear warnings of the health risks of smoking also indicated that fat consumption as such was not a health risk. The massive Hammond Report, which surveyed well over a million subjects, was presented to the American Medical Association's Annual Meeting on December 4, 1963. The surprise finding in the Hammond Report was that the more times per week that subjects ate fried foods—and keep in mind that in the early 1960s most frying used animal fats—the lower their death rates. This is virtually the same as concluding that the more saturated fats that were eaten, the longer the subjects lived. The Hammond Report was deemed authoritative when it came to the health hazards of cigarette smoking, but completely ignored when it came to the issue of dietary fats. Its very strong epidemiological evidence that dietary fat consumption was not linked to heart disease did not fit the current medical model of that time.

On June 15, 1993, the results of the third National Health and Nutrition Examination Study were released by the National Center for Health Statistics. These results showed that the average blood cholesterol reading for American adults has declined from 220 milligrams per deciliter (mg/dL) in 1960–1962 to 205 mg/dL for the period 1988–1991. Most news accounts have linked this decline in cholesterol readings to the decline in death rates from cardiovascular disease (CVD) over the same thirty-year period. Not mentioned in such stories is the success over the last three decades of modern medical interventive techniques (discussed above). Also not mentioned is the striking difference in the statistical picture between the United States and France. American males have an average cholesterol reading of 209 mg/dL, perhaps lower, and a CVD death rate of 197 per 100,000. French males have a much higher cholesterol average of 230 mg/dL, yet they also have a far lower CVD death rate of only 78 per 100,000. In addition, we should not forget that the French continue to smoke at a rate far above the current American norm.[13]

It will be much easier to understand the nature of the confusion regarding cholesterol if the following points are kept in mind: First, the body itself manufactures two-thirds or more of its own cholesterol, and it can do this even from a diet consisting mostly of carbohydrates. Some quite small percentage of the populace is genetically disposed to produce far too much cholesterol, but this fraction does not include the vast majority of us. Second, cholesterol is the base for a great many of the body's key hormones and it is found in all cell membranes. Third, a growing number of researchers now accept that cardiovascular disease may be a subclinical sign of problems involving insulin regulation and/or free-radical damage. Finally, in all the major population studies done on cholesterol, it was usually next to impossible to lower blood cholesterol by dietary means unless the subjects also lost excess weight.

This last point is, of course, the key. Obesity, especially if characterized by excess abdominal fat (which often indicates lowered thyroid function) can increase the risk of heart disease by as much as 300 percent. If we factor in the problems caused by excess weight and add to this the modern American tendency to rely upon canned and frozen foods (which through processing lose almost all of their intrinsic antioxidants and many of the naturally present vitamins and minerals), then it becomes much simpler to explain why cardiovascular disease is such a problem in the United States at the end of the twentieth century.

Does this mean that diet and blood cholesterol levels do not matter? Not at all. Individuals with cholesterol levels above 200 and with bad HDL-to-LDL ratios may be faced with elevated health risks. As a short-term therapeutic diet, the very-low-fat Pritikin Diet discussed in Chapter 5 has proven quite successful for many individuals. Likewise, cholesterol-lowering regimens using niacin, oat bran, and the like (see Robert E. Kowalski's *The 8-Week Cholesterol Cure*) have their place in therapeutics.

The trick is to avoid blaming the messenger. If high serum (blood) levels of LDLs in fact represent the body's attempt to compensate for a lack of antioxidants, then lowering cholesterol levels through heroic dietary measures and drug intervention is a false victory. If high cholesterol levels merely mark the presence of cholesterol-containing hormones associated with the body's response to stress, then the real answer is to slow down, not to starve the body of the building blocks for hormones. Finally, if high LDL cholesterol levels, and especially high triglyceride levels, are the result of insulin resistance and a diet high in sucrose, fructose, and refined carbohydrates and low in vitamins and minerals such as chromium, then the permanent solution is to stabilize blood sugar levels. Remember, the Atkins Diet (high protein, high fat, low carbohydrate) also is successful as a therapeutic diet.

NUTRIENTS CONTROL CHOLESTEROL AND HEART DISEASE

Now, it should be recognized that conclusions such as those presented in the Hammond Report have not been thoroughly examined by the American medical research community. Only recently have significant new ways of approaching the issue of heart disease been widely entertained. Two of these deserve some attention here. The first is that of excessive iron in the diet, and the second and related question is that of the adequacy of antioxidants in the diet. Let us begin with the role of iron in heart and other diseases.

Iron is very important in human nutrition, and it is perhaps the most widely supplemented mineral in everyday foods. However, as with other minerals, the important thing is to get the right amount. Too much iron in the diets of children, men, and postmenopausal women has been linked to increases in a wide variety of diseases, and the common practice of "fortifying" American foods with iron has been harshly condemned by a number of leading medical authorities.[14]

Recently, the journal *Circulation* reviewed evidence showing that the extremely high risk of heart attacks characteristic of men in eastern Finland reflects not just high blood cholesterol levels, but also very high levels of iron.[15] As the editor of the journal pointed out, the connection is now being made between findings of this type and the dramatic increase in heart disease observed in women following menopause.

The argument being put forward by medical researchers is this: Men, unless they are involved in very heavy physical labor or endurance athletics, tend to readily collect iron in the body since they do not excrete it regularly. After women stop menstruating, they, too, begin to collect iron in their tissues. Excess iron is known to interfere with the heart muscle's contractions. However, the primary danger posed by excess iron is freeradical damage. Iron acts as a catalyst to oxidative processes, and in excess it promotes the oxidation of LDLs, also known as the "bad" lipids. The damaged LDLs settle into the walls of arteries and narrow them. In careful studies it has been learned that men who had high blood cholesterol levels who also had the highest levels of iron suffered twice the heart attack rate of the normal population. Furthermore, there is some evidence that those most at risk are individuals who are genetically predisposed to store iron.[16]

In addition to infectious diseases and heart disease, cancer has been linked to the excessive consumption of iron, especially by men. The likely mechanism is the same suggested for heart disease, that is, some sort of free-radical damage encouraged by excess iron in the tissues.[17] Still other diseases, such as arthritis, similarly may be caused, or at least triggered, by high tissue levels of iron.

In brief, most men, especially if sedentary, and postmenopausal women probably should avoid additional sources of iron since this mineral is already added to many foods. However, it remains well established that premenopausal women and athletes may require supplemental iron.[18]

The role of antioxidants in preventing heart disease is thus indicated by studies involving iron. However, the usefulness of antioxidants is far more general than that. Vitamin C has long been known to help control oxidation of LDL, and therefore to help prevent its deposit onto arterial walls (atherosclerosis). Indeed, a UCLA study published in 1992 surveying more than 11,000 subjects showed that an increased intake of vitamin C was associated with a 50 percent reduction in death from heart disease and a more than six-year prolongation of life.

In 1989, Dr. Linus Pauling discovered that a protein formed in the liver from LDL serves as a substitute for vitamin C when the latter's serum levels are low. Adequate levels of vitamin C prevent the deposit of this protein onto artery walls. The implication is that atherosclerosis is essentially a form of scurvy. Subsequently in 1991, Dr. Pauling and Dr. Matthias Rath published an article in the *Journal of Orthomolecular Medicine* that detailed the causative mechanism of cardiovascular disease.[19] Also in 1991, a combination of vitamin C and the amino acid lysine was used to improve heart function and to overcome angina.[20] Lysine serves as a precursor to the synthesis of L-carnitine by the body, and it also serves to bind the very protein that Drs. Pauling and Rath argue leads to the formation of arterial plaques. The use of the combination of lysine and vitamin C offers the theoretical possibility of reversing this buildup, and it has been shown to do so in one case.

The protective effect of nutrients, of course, is not limited to vitamin C. Similar protection has been shown to exist from vitamin E, beta-carotene, copper, magnesium, manganese, zinc, and other such vitamins and minerals, which either act as antioxidants and cell-membrane stabilizers themselves or act as precursors to the body's own enzyme antioxidants, such as superoxide dismutase (SOD).[21]

"DISEASES OF CIVILIZATION"

Coronary heart disease, as is true of adult-onset diabetes, extensive tooth decay, and many other degenerative afflictions, might rightly be called a disease of civilization.[22] These health problems often take decades to become manifest, and therefore it is easy to overlook their relationship to a diet of refined and nutrient-poor foods. Excessive weight gain, likewise, can take years to become a seemingly permanent part of our lives and a source of concern. Certainly the damage to the body's regulatory mechanisms can take place long before the pounds begin to accumulate. However, there are some highly visible signs of impending health problems that usually are apparent long before we can speak of heart disease or diabetes or even a "weight problem." Perhaps the most significant of these indications of future problems is the health of our teeth, and we should spend a little time in closing to consider just why this should be so.

We Americans suffer so ubiquitously from dental cavities that we seldom realize that not all the world suffers with us. Various brands of toothpaste are advertised nightly on TV, and brushing, flossing, and gargling with mouthwash are routinely touted to solve all dental problems. Yet bad teeth follow the adoption of a Western diet, with sugary British and American diets always at the fore. What is not often realized (because it is hidden by the successes of our medical *intervention* in cases of disease, as opposed to our medical *prevention* of disease) is that bad teeth and degenerative diseases usually are found together. As one classic text, *Diet and Disease,* puts it regarding coronary artery disease, obesity, diabetes, and hyperglyceridemia:

> Dental caries is [sic] intimately associated with the geographic incidence of these "diseases of civilization." Doctor Fred L. Losee . . . has observed a strong geographic correlation between digestive tract cancer and dental decay. As was noted for coronary artery disease, obesity, diabetes, and gout, the ingestion of large quantities of refined carbohydrates is causally related to the carious lesion. It has been emphasized that this type of overnutrition may be a potentiating factor in a variety of chronic conditions.
>
> A pathological oral finding which has been observed to occur in relation to coronary artery disease is dental calculus (tartar) . . . it appears that the rate of deposition is positively correlated with the personal and family history of coronary artery disease.[23]

Virtually everyone is aware of the clear relationship between the consumption of sugar and tooth decay. However, the quite surprising finding around the world is that the consumption of sugar cane itself does *not* lead to cavities! Cane workers in South Africa who chewed four stalks of cane a day had better-than-average teeth.[24] Similarly in laboratory experiments, mixtures of saliva and sugar, and saliva and cane juice were tested on teeth that had been removed but that had no cavities. Weeks later half of the teeth in the sugar had been demineralized, whereas those in the cane juice had not.[25]

This same contrast between refined and raw sugar exists with respect to diabetes. In a province of eastern South Africa known as the Natal, diabetes among the cane cutters, who consume large amounts of the raw cane themselves, is virtually unknown, whereas there are very high correlations between the consumption of refined sugar and deaths from diabetes.[26] In another revealing instance, during the 1920s with the construction of the Panama Canal, some five thousand workers from the Dominican Republic were examined—these were people who had eaten cane since childhood—and no cases of diabetes were found. On the other hand, the wealthy Spanish of the area, who ate refined sugar in large amounts, were extremely prone to diabetes.[27]

Diabetes and obesity, in most cases, are closely related, so the importance of this example to the dieter is clear. The vitamins, minerals, and other unknown factors in the raw cane made the consumption of it in large amounts a nonissue as far as dental and general health were concerned. Nevertheless, as a refined product, sugar is a deadly enemy to both, for it radically disturbs the metabolism of minerals, insulin, and lipids.

As we have seen, most of the same processes that lead to excessive weight gain also lead to cardiovascular and similar problems. It should also be pointed out that obesity is linked to fatty deposits in the aorta and coronary arteries even in young adults and children.[28]

Nutrient-rich diets high in fiber, in vitamins and minerals, in special "health" foods (for example, spirulina, whole grains such as barley and spelt, and so on), and in quality fats are not associated with any of the diseases of civilization. Lifestyles that include moderate exercise, such as thirty minutes of brisk walking three times per week, likewise are not associated with modern degenerative illnesses.

Concluding Thoughts

The first edition of this book came out a decade ago. In the intervening years, much of what has been advocated within its pages has become accepted by mainstream, mass-market vitamin companies. Today we have One-a-Day multivitamins with metabolism enhancers and similar products appearing everywhere. All of these are presented as being "new," but we should not forget our roots. More than forty years ago, Roger J. Williams, the discoverer of many of the vitamins, published a book called *Biochemical Individuality* (Wiley, 1956), in which he argued that:

- There is no such thing as the average person.

- Some of us are better than others at detoxifying drugs and chemicals.

- Some people are more prone to diabetes than are others.

- Low-fat diets cause some individuals to gain weight.

- One person needs higher levels of nutrients than another to maintain health.

These points are as true today as they were in 1956. In dieting, as in other areas of health, each of us needs to select a program that matches our own particular physiology, habits, and circumstances.

The first step is to get a handle on why you—not your neighbors—have gained weight. Return to Chapter 5. Look through this chapter to isolate those aspects of diet, exercise, and other habits that have led to your unwanted weight gain. For instance, if stress is a factor in your weight gain, then metabolic stimulants may be short-term fixes that, in the long run, make your weight problem worse. If wretched dietary habits are to blame—and you likely already know this means you!—then not only a change in diet, but also nutrients that support proper metabolism may be in order.

The second step is to decide on a realistic goal. Again, not the goal that is right for your neighbor, your son or daughter, or some fashion model, but the goal that is right for you with your body and your genes.

The third step involves learning what you reasonably can expect from supplements and whether you have one or more special conditions that need to be addressed. For example, conquering Syndrome X will not in and of itself necessarily make you lean. Nevertheless, it is an absolutely essential requirement for getting lean and staying there if you are insulin resistant.

Next, carefully familiarize yourself with the many nutrients that are available. Some may be of interest to you, but others may not. However, even those items that do not match your dieting needs may still be of interest. Coenzyme Q_{10}, for instance, only helps a relatively small percentage of individuals lose weight, but it helps many more who have gum problems or need to support immune functioning.

Finally, do not be afraid to experiment. Give any set of supplements you try a chance to deliver, which usually means a two- or three-month trial. Many of the supplements can be used together, but some are alternatives. Be clear as to which is the case. If after a good trial, a supplement does not work for you, try to find out why and, if necessary, use a different tact. It is, after all, your health, your life.

Nutritional Analysis of Foods

The following table is designed to be used in conjunction with Chapter 4. Those dieters who wish to practice food coupling will find that weight loss is greater with larger protein portions, as indicated in the text, coupled with more vegetables. The combination of carbohydrates and fats, to the contrary, tends to lead to the storage of calories. Therefore, if in this table the amount of fat for a given food is high, that food preferably should be eaten with protein and at least one portion of vegetables, and preferably two portions. The numbers below, for the most part, are based on cooked portions and are approximations that reflect average conditions. Finally, although in this age of "supersized" portions many of us need reminders regarding reasonable serving sizes, dieters should not fixate on total calories. Over the long run, it is a more successful strategy to avoid bad food combinations and to eat foods that provide plenty of filling bulk, such as vegetables and soups, than it is to pay too much attention to calories.

Food	Quantity	Calories (grams)	Protein (grams)	Carbohydrate (grams)	Fat (grams)
Dairy and Eggs					
Butter	1 tablespoon	100	—	—	11
Cheddar cheese	1/2 cup	226	14	1	19
Cottage cheese	1/2 cup	100	14	4	2
Eggs	2	150	12	—	12
Egg yolks	2	120	6	—	10
Ice cream	1 cup	300	6	29	18
Milk (nonfat)	1 quart	360	36	52	—
Swiss cheese	1 slice	105	7	—	8

Food	Quantity	Calories (grams)	Protein (grams)	Carbohydrate (grams)	Fat (grams)
Yogurt (nonfat)	1 cup	120	8	13	4
Meats/Poultry/Fish					
Ground beef	3 ounces (oz)	185	24	—	10
Roast beef	3 oz	390	16	—	36
Steak (lean)	3 oz	220	24	—	12
Chicken	3 oz	185	23	—	9
Duck	3 oz	370	16	—	28
Lamb	4 oz	480	24	—	12
Pork	3$\frac{1}{2}$ oz	200	16	—	21
Ham	4 oz	340	26	—	26
Turkey	3$\frac{1}{2}$ oz	265	27	—	15
Veal	3 oz	185	23	—	9
Cod	3$\frac{1}{2}$ oz	170	25	—	5
Halibut	3$\frac{1}{2}$ oz	182	26	—	8
Lobster	3 oz	92	18	—	1
Swordfish	3 oz	180	27	—	6
Salmon	3 oz	120	17	—	5
Tuna	3 oz	170	25	—	7
Vegetables					
Artichoke	1 large	25	2	10	—
Asparagus	6 spears	18	1	3	—
Broccoli	1 cup	45	5	8	—
Brussels sprouts	1 cup	60	6	12	—
Cabbage	1 cup	36	1	9	—
Cauliflower	1 cup	30	3	6	—
Celery	1 cup	20	1	4	—
Corn	1 cup	170	5	41	—
Cucumber	1 cup	6	—	1	—
Eggplant	1 cup	30	2	9	—
Green beans	1 cup	25	1	6	—
Kidney beans	1 cup	230	15	42	—

Food	Quantity	Calories (grams)	Protein (grams)	Carbohydrate (grams)	Fat (grams)
Lettuce	1/4 head	14	1	2	–
Lima beans	1 cup	140	16	48	–
Mushrooms	1/2 cup	12	2	4	–
Navy beans	1 cup	250	11	37	–
Onions	1 cup	80	2	18	–
Potatoes (mashed)	1 cup	230	4	28	12
Soybeans	1 cup	260	22	20	11
Spinach	1 cup	26	3	3	–
Squash, summer	1 cup	35	1	8	–
Sweet potato	1 medium	155	2	36	1
Tomato	1 medium	30	1	6	–
Fruits					
Apple	1 medium	70	–	18	–
Apricots	3 medium	55	1	14	–
Avocado	1 large	370	4	12	36
Banana	1 medium	85	1	23	–
Cantaloupe	1/2 medium	40	1	9	–
Grapefruit	1/2 medium	50	1	14	–
Grapes	1 cup	70	1	16	–
Olives	10	72	1	3	10
Orange	1 medium	60	2	16	–
Papaya	1 medium	150	2	36	–
Peach	1 medium	35	1	10	–
Plum	1 medium	30	–	7	–
Raisins	1/2 cup	230	2	62	–
Strawberries	1 cup	54	–	12	–
Watermelon	1 slice	120	2	29	1
Bread/Cereal/Grains					
Bran flakes	1 cup	117	3	3	2
Bread, rye	1 slice	55	2	12	–
Bread, wheat	1 slice	55	2	11	1

Food	Quantity	Calories (grams)	Protein (grams)	Carbohydrate (grams)	Fat (grams)
Macaroni	1 cup	155	5	32	1
Noodles	1 cup	200	7	37	2
Oatmeal	1 cup	150	5	26	3
Buckwheat pancakes	4	250	7	28	9
Brown rice	1 cup	748	15	154	3
Roll, wheat	1	102	4	20	1
Spaghetti with meat sauce	1 cup	285	13	35	10
Nuts					
Almonds	1/2 cup	425	13	13	38
Cashews	1/2 cup	281	12	20	32
Peanut butter (unsalted)	1/3 cup	284	13	8	24
Peanuts, natural	1/3 cup	290	13	9	25
Pecans, roasted	1/2 cup	343	5	7	35
Walnuts	1/2 cup	325	7	8	32
Misc.					
Olive, soy, safflower, corn oil	1 tablespoon	110	—	—	12

Notes

Introduction: Beyond Calorie Counting

1. "Methods for voluntary weight loss and control," NIH Technology Assessment Conference Panel, *Annals of Internal Medicine* 1992 June;1165(11): 942–949.

2: The Anti-Fat Nutrients

1. PA Southorn and G Powis, "Free radicals in medicine. I. Chemical nature and biologic reactions," *Mayo Clin Proc* 1988 Apr;63(4):381–9; PA Southorn and G Powis, "Free radicals in medicine. II. Involvement in human disease," *Mayo Clin Proc* 1988 Apr;63(4):390–408.

2. L Cremer, A Herold, D Avram, G Szegli, "A purified green barley extract with modulatory properties upon TNF alpha and ROS released by human specialised cells isolated from RA patients," *Roum Arch Microbiol Immunol* 1998 Jul–Dec;57(3–4):231–42; YM Yu, WC Chang, et al., "Effects of young barley leaf extract and antioxidative vitamins on LDL oxidation and free radical scavenging activities in type 2 diabetes," *Diabetes Metab* 2002 Apr;28(2):107–14.

3. L Packer, et al., "Alpha-lipoic acid as a biological antioxidant," *Free Radical Biology & Medicine* 1995;19:227–250.

4. Jean Barilla, ed., *The Antioxidants*, vol. 1, *The Nutrition Superbook* (Keats Publishing, 1995); DG Williams, "Cleaning house," *Alternatives* 1992 Jul;4, 12:97–100.

5. Sandra Goodman, *Vitamin C: The Master Nutrient* (Keats Publishing, 1991); M Meydani, "Nutrition interventions in aging and age-associated disease," *Proc Nutr Soc* 2002 May;61(2):165–71.

6. W Rumpler, et al., "Oolong tea increases metabolic rate and fat oxidation in men," *J Nutr* 2001 Nov;131(11):2848–52; M Yang, C Wang, and H Chen, "Green, oolong and black tea extracts modulate lipid metabolism in hyperlipidemia rats fed high-sucrose diet," *J Nutr Biochem* 2001 Jan;12(1):14–20; A Dulloo, et al., "Efficacy of a green tea extract rich in catechin polyphenols and caffeine in increasing 24-h energy expenditure and fat oxidation in humans," *Am J of Clin Nutr* 1999;70:1040–45.

7. KV Ingold and GW Burton, "Bioavailability on various forms of vitamin E," Henkel Vitamin E Conference (1991).

8. KS Williamson, et al., "The nitration product 5-nitro-gamma-tocopherol is increased in the Alzheimer brain," *Nitric Oxide* 2002 Mar;6(2):221–7.

9. Leon Chaitow, *Amino Acids in Therapy* (Healing Arts Press, 1988), 79–81.

10. EC Opara, et al., "L-glutamine supplementation of a high fat diet reduces body weight and attenuates hyperglycemia and hyperinsulinemia in C57BL/6J mice," *J Nutr* 1996 Jan;126(1):273–9.

11. For the anorectic properties of wall germander see *International Journal of Crude Drug Research* 1989 Dec;27(4): 201–10.

12. Alfred Goodman Gilman, Louis S Goodman, et al., eds., *Goodman and Gilman's The Pharmacological Basis of Therapeutics*, 6th ed. (Macmillan, 1980), 253 and 653; Durk Pearson and Sandy Shaw, *The Life Extension Weight Loss Program* (Doubleday, 1986), 109ff.

13. AJ Hill, et al., "Oral administration of proteinase inhibitor II from potatoes reduces energy intake in man," *Physiol Behav* 1990 Aug;48(2):abstract 241–6.

14. TA Spiegel, C Hubert, SR Peikin, University of Medicine & Dentistry of New Jersey, "Effect of a premeal beverage containing a protease inhibitor from potatoes on satiety in dieting overweight women," *Obesity Research* Nov 1999;7(1):abstract.

15. AJ Hawthorne and RF Butterwick, "The satiating effect of a diet containing jojoba meal (*Simmondsia chinensis*) in dogs," *J of Nutr* 1998;128:2669S–2670S.

16. T Andersen and J Fogh, "Weight loss and delayed gastric emptying following a South American herbal preparation in overweight patients." *J Hum Nutr Diet* 2001 Jun;14 (3):243–50.

17. On spirulina, see Christopher Hills, ed., *The Secrets of Spirulina: Medical Discoveries of Japanese Doctors,* trans. Robert Wargo (University of the Trees Press, 1980). See the discussions of nutrient partitioning on pages 31 and 134.

18. C Gemma, et al., "Diets enriched in foods with high antioxidant activity reverse age-induced decreases in cerebellar beta-adrenergic function and increases in proinflammatory cytokines, *J Neurosci* 2002 Jul 15;22(14):6114–6120.

19. VK Mazo, et al., "Effect of biologically active food additives containing autolysate of baker's yeast and spirulina on intestinal permeability in an experiment," *Vopr Pitan* 1999;68(1):17–9.

20. C Gonzalez de Rivera, et al., "Preventive effect of *Spirulina maxima* on the fatty liver induced by a fructose-rich diet in the rat, a preliminary report," *Life Sci* 1993;53(1):57–61.

21. K Iwata, T Inayama, and T Kato, "Effects of *Spirulina platensis* on plasma lipoprotein lipase activity in fructose-induced hyperlipidemic rats," *J Nutr Sci Vitaminol* (Tokyo) 1990 Apr;36(2):165–71.

22. C Cangiano, et al., "Effects of 5-hydroxytryptophan on eating behavior and adherence to dietary prescriptions in obese adult subjects," *Adv Exp Med Biol* 1991;294:591–3.

23. C Cangiano, et al., "Effects of oral 5-hydroxy-tryptophan on energy intake and macronutrient selection in non-insulin dependent diabetic patients," *Int J Obes Relat Metab Disord* 1998 Jul;22(7):648–54.

24. C Cangiano, et al., "Eating behavior and adherence to dietary prescriptions in obese adult subjects treated with 5-hydroxytryptophan," *Am J Clin Nutr* 1992 Nov;56(5):863–7.

25. GS Kelly, "*Rhodiola rosea*: a possible plant adaptogen," *Altern Med Rev* 2001 Jun;6(3):293–302.

26. Durk Pearson and Sandy Shaw, *The Life Extension Weight Loss Program* (Doubleday, 1986), 109ff.; Leon Chaitow, *Amino Acids in Therapy,* (Healing Arts Press, 1988), 58–61, 77–78.

27. L Abenhaim, et al., "Appetite-suppressant drugs and the risk of primary pulmonary hypertension," International Primary Pulmonary Hypertension Study Group, *N Engl J Med* 1996 Aug 29;335(9):609–16.

28. JT Favreau, et al., "Severe hepatotoxicity associated with the dietary supplement LipoKinetix," *Ann Intern Med* 2002 Apr 16;136(8):590–5.

29. J Liu, et al., "Memory loss in old rats is associated with brain mitochondrial decay and RNA/DNA oxidation: partial reversal by feeding acetyl-L-carnitine and/or R-alpha-lipoic acid," *Proc Natl Acad Sci USA* 2002 Feb 19;99(4):2356–61; TM Hagen, et al., "Feeding acetyl-L-carnitine and lipoic acid to old rats significantly improves metabolic function while decreasing oxidative stress," *Proc Natl Acad Sci USA* 2002 Feb 19;99(4):1870–5.

30. MF McCarty, "Hepatothermic therapy of obesity: rationale and an inventory of resources," *Med Hypotheses* 2001 Sept;57(3):324–36; RG Villani, et al., "L-Carnitine supplementation combined with aerobic training does not promote weight loss in moderately obese women," *Int J Sport Nutr Exerc Metab* 2000 Jun;10(2):199–207; YS Cha, et al., "Effects of carnitine coingested caffeine on carnitine metabolism and endurance capacity in athletes," *J Nutr Sci Vitaminol* (Tokyo) 2001 Dec;47(6):378–84; ME Mitchell, "Carnitine metabolism in human subjects. I. Normal metabolism," *Am J Clin Nutr* 1978 Feb;31(2):293–306.

31. Jeffrey Bland, *Octacosanol, Carnitine, and Other "Accessory" Nutrients* (Keats Publishing, 1982).

32. P Hahn, "Serum carnitine levels and hepatic and adipose tissue carnitine transferases in obese mice," *Nutrition Research* 1981;1:93–99; AT Davis, PG Davis, SD Phinney, et al., "Plasma and urinary carnitine of obese subjects on very-low-calorie diets," *J Am Coll Nutr* 1990 Jun;9(3):261–4.

33. V Bettini, et al., "Potentiating effect of L-carnitine on the in-vitro methacholine-induced relaxation of massenteric arteries," in *Drugs in Competitive Athletics,* ed. JR Shipe (Blackwell, 1991), 107–113.

34. SA Center, et al., "The clinical and metabolic effects of rapid weight loss in obese pet cats and the influence of supplemental oral L-carnitine," *J Vet Intern Med* 2000 Nov/Dec;14(6):598–608.

35. JW Daily III and DS Sachan, "Choline supplementation alters carnitine homeostasis in humans and guinea pigs," *J Nutr* 1995 Jul;125(7):1938–44.

36. A Khan, et al., "Insulin potentiating factor and chromium content of selected foods and spices," *Biologic Trace Element Research* 1990;24:183–188.

37. The best readily accessible recent review of all the pertinent data on chromium is Richard A Passwater, *Chromium Picolinate* (Keats Publishing, 1992). On the virtues of chromium polynicotinate (ChromMate), see K Olin, et al., "Comparative retention/absorption of chromium (Cr) from Cr chloride, Cr nicotinate and Cr picolinate in a rat model," 33rd Annual Meeting of the American College of Nutrition, October 10, 1992. Chrome-Mate is absorbed and retained roughly three times better than is chromium picolinate. However, bioavailability was not assessed.

38. Passwater, *Chromium Picolinate*, passim; JR Roeback Jr, et al., "Effects of chromium supplementation on serum high-density lipoprotein cholesterol levels in men taking beta-blockers," *Ann Intern Med* 1991 Dec 15;115(12):917–24. This randomized, controlled trial reported that chromium supplementation raised HDL levels in patients whose levels have been driven artificially and dangerously lower by diuretics and beta-blockers. Also see the informative discussion in Elson M Haas, *Staying Healthy with Nutrition* (Celestial Arts, 1992), 187–190.

39. Haas, *Staying Healthy with Nutrition*, 187.

40. CE Heyliger, AG Tahiliani, and JH McNeill, "Effect of vanadate on elevated blood glucose and depressed cardiac performance of diabetic rats," *Science* 1985 Mar 22;227 (4693):1474–7.

41. JZ Meyerovitch, et al., "Oral administration of vanadate normalizes blood glucose levels in streptozotocin-treated rats," *J Biol Chem* 1987;262:6658–6662; DJ Paulson, et al., "Effects of vanadate on in vivo reactivity to norepinephrine in diabetic rats," *J Pharmacol Exp Therapy* 1987;240:529–534.

42. MA Abou-Seif, "Oxidative stress of vanadium-mediated oxygen free radical generation stimulated by aluminium on human erythrocytes," *Ann Clin Biochem* 1998 Mar;35 (pt 2):254–60.

43. AK Srivastava, "Anti-diabetic and toxic effects of vanadium compounds," *Mol Cell Biochem* 2000 Mar;206(1–2):177–82.

44. ZK Atta-Ur-Rahman, "Medicinal plants with hypoglycemic activity," *J Ethnopharmacol* 1989 Jun;26(1):1–55.

45. V Shanbhag, "*Gymnema sylvestre:* a vedic wonder-drug for diabetes," *Health World* 1990 Jan/Feb:34ff.

46. H Katsukawa, T Imoto, and Y Ninomiya, "Induction of salivary gurmarin-binding proteins in rats fed gymnema-containing diets," *Chem Senses* 1999 Aug;24(4):387–92.

47. SJ Persaud, H Al-Majed, A Raman, and PM Jones, "*Gymnema sylvestre* stimulates insulin release in vitro by increased membrane permeability," *J Endocrinol* 1999 Nov;163(2):207–12.

48. WV Judy, et al., "Antidiabetic activity of a standardized extract (Glucosol) from *Lagerstroemia speciosa* leaves in Type II diabetics. A dose-dependence study," *J Ethnopharmacol* 2003 Jul;87(1):115–7.

49. T Kakuda, I Sakane, T Takihara, Y Ozaki, H Takeuchi, and M Kuroyanagi, "Hypoglycemic effect of extracts from *Lagerstroemia speciosa* L. leaves in genetically diabetic KK-AY mice," *Biosci Biotechnol Biochem* 1996 Feb;60(2):204–8.

50. C Murakami, K Myoga, R Kasai, K Ohtani, T Kurokawa, S Ishibashi, F Dayrit, WG Padolina, and K Yamasaki, "Screening of plant constituents for effect on glucose transport activity in Ehrlich ascites tumour cells," *Chem Pharm Bull* (Tokyo) 1993 Dec;41(12):2129–31.

51. WV Judy, "Glucosol balances blood sugar levels," Natural Products Expo West March 23, 2000 (presentation).

52. Michael Colgan ("Vanadium: the bottom line," *Muscular Development* 1992 Mar:14, 168) argues that vanadium in all its forms is toxic in any effective dosage. Evidence shows

that vanadium given in the water supply to rats causes extreme diarrhea and death from electrolyte loss. However, these are not the classic symptoms of poisoning. The type of supplementation used may be at fault for these results, that is, through the water supply. Toxicity in any reasonable dosage has not been reported for vanadyl sulfate in human subjects. In fact, vanadium has enjoyed extensive use in treating a variety of human ailments with few side effects. Dosages of above 20 mg taken for extended periods of time may lead to mild readily reversable gastrointestinal irritation. For a complete review see: HA Schroeder, et al., "Abnormal trace metals in man—vanadium," *J Chron Disease* 1963; 16:1047–1071; and JH McNeill, et al., "Bis(maltolato)oxyvanadium(IV) is a potent insulin mimic," *J Med Chem* 1992;35:1489–1491. As noted in the text, some informal studies have suggested that the upper limit of an effective dosage is far below that of toxicity. There is no reason for ingesting dosages that exceed such an upper limit; therefore, nutritional levels of intake remain within the margins of safety. Cases of active diabetes may prove to be exceptions to this because in such instances effective dosage levels are much higher than in nondiabetics.

53. S Sugiyama, et al., "Antioxidative effect of coenzyme Q_{10}," *Experientia* 1980;36: 1002–1003.

54. Emile G Bliznakov and Gerald L Hunt, *The Miracle Nutrient Coenzyme CoQ10* (Bantam Books, 1986), 50–154, citing the Belgian studies of Dr. Luc Van Gaal and his colleagues.

55. MF McCarty, "Toward practical prevention of type 2 diabetes," *Med Hypotheses* 2000 May;54(5):786–93.

56. K Folkers, et al., eds. *Biomedical and Clinical Aspects of Coenzyme Q* (Elsevier Science Publishers, 1991), 513–520.

57. FL Rosenfeldt, et al., "Coenzyme Q_{10} protects the aging heart against stress: studies in rats, human tissues, and patients," *Ann N Y Acad Sci* 2002 Apr;959:355–9, discussion 463–5. See the general review in Brian Leibovitz, "Coenzyme Q," *Nutrition & Fitness* 1991; X(3–4): 47–48.

58. SR Thomas, J Neuzil, and R Stocker, "Cosupplementation with coenzyme Q prevents the prooxidant effect of alpha-tocopherol and increases the resistance of LDL to transition metal-dependent oxidation initiation," *Arterioscler Thromb Vasc Biol* 1996 May;16 (5):687–96.

59. CC Miller, Y Park, MW Pariza, and ME Cook, "Feeding conjugated linoleic acid to animals partially overcomes catabolic responses due to endotoxin injection," *Biochem Biophys Res Commun* 1994 Feb 15;198(3):1107–12.

60. RJ Nicolosi, et al., "Decreased aortic early atherosclerosis in hypercholesterolemic hamsters fed oleic acid-rich TriSun oil compared to linoleic acid-rich sunflower oil," *J Nutr Biochem* 2002 Jul;13(7):392–402. See also P Benito, et al., "The effect of conjugated linoleic acid on plasma lipoproteins and tissue fatty acid composition in humans," *Lipids* 2001 Mar;36(3):229–36.

61. ME Cook, CC Miller, Y Park, and M Pariza, "Immune modulation by altered nutrient metabolism: nutritional control of immune-induced growth depression," *Poult Sci* 1993 Jul;72(7):1301–5.

62. GI Stangl, "Conjugated linoleic acids exhibit a strong fat-to-lean partitioning effect, reduce serum VLDL lipids and redistribute tissue lipids in food-restricted rats," *J Nutr* 2000 May;130(5):1140–6.

63. AH Terpstra, et al., "The decrease in body fat in mice fed conjugated linoleic acid is due to increases in energy expenditure and energy loss in the excreta," *J Nutr* 2002 May;132(5):940–5.

64. U Riserus, L Berglund, and B Vessby, "Conjugated linoleic acid (CLA) reduced abdominal adipose tissue in obese middle-aged men with signs of the metabolic syndrome: a randomised controlled trial," *Int J Obes Relat Metab Disord* 2001 Aug;25(8):1129–35.

65. H Blankson, et al., "Conjugated linoleic acid reduces body fat mass in overweight and obese humans," *J Nutr* 2000 Dec;130(12):2943–8.

66. MW Pariza, Y Park, and ME Cook, "Conjugated linoleic acid and the control of cancer and obesity," *Toxicol Sci* 1999 Dec;52(suppl 2):107–10.

67. SF Chin, et al., "Conjugated linoleic acid is a growth factor for rats as shown by enhanced weight gain and improved feed efficiency," *J of Nutr* 1994;124:2344–2349.

68. T Ringbom, U Huss, A Stenholm, S Flock, L Skattebol, P Perera, and L Bohlin, "Cox-2 inhibitory effects of naturally occurring and modified fatty acids," *J Nat Prod* 2001 Jun;64(6):745–9.

69. J Whitaker, "New hope on obesity and diabetes," *Health & Healing* 1992 Oct;2(11):4–5, 8.

70. M Davidson, et al., "Safety and pharmacokinetic study with escalating doses of 3-acetyl-7-oxo-dehydroepiandrosterone in healthy male volunteers," *Clin Invest Med* 2000 Oct;23(5):300–10.

71. Ibid; DL Coleman, et al., "Therapeutic effects of dehydroepiandrosterone (DHEA) in diabetic mice," *Diabetes* 1982;31:830–833; "Effect of genetic background on the therapeutic effects of dehydroepiandrosterone (DHEA) in diabetes-obesity mutants in aged normal mice," *Diabetes* 1984;33:26; "Antiobesity effects of etiocholanolones in diabetes (db), viable yellow (Avy), and normal mice," *Endrocrinology* 1985;117:2279–2283.

72. AA Tagliaferro, et al., "The effect of dehydroepiandrosterone (DHEA) on calorie intake, body weight, and resting metabolism," *Federation Proceeding* 1983;42:326(abstract 201).

73. HD Danenberg, A Ben-Yehuda, Z Zakay-Rones, DJ Gross, and G Friedman, "Dehydroepiandrosterone treatment is not beneficial to the immune response to influenza in elderly subjects," *J Clin Endocrinol Metab* 1997 Sept;82(9):2911-4; A Ben-Yehuda, HD Danenberg, Z Zakay-Rones, DJ Gross, and G Friedman, "The influence of sequential annual vaccination and of DHEA administration on the efficacy of the immune response to influenza vaccine in the elderly," *Mech Ageing Dev* 1998 May 15;102(2-3):299-306.

74. SS Yen, AJ Morales, and O Khorram, "Replacement of DHEA in aging men and women. Potential remedial effects," *Ann N Y Acad Sci* 1995 Dec 29;774:128-42; RF van Vollenhoven, "Dehydroepiandrosterone for the treatment of systemic lupus erythematosus," *Expert Opin Pharmacother* 2002 Jan;3(1):23-31; S Legrain and L Girard, "Pharmacology and therapeutic effects of dehydroepiandrosterone in older subjects," *Drugs Aging* 2003;20(13):94.

75. KS Usiskin, et al., "Lack of effect of dehydroepiandrosterone in obese men," *Int J Obes* 1990 May;14(5):457–63; JE Nestler, et al., "Suppression of serum dehydroepiandrosterone sulfate levels by insulin: an evaluation of possible mechanisms," *J Clin Endocrinol Metab* 1989 Nov;69(5):1040-6; AJ Morales, JJ Nolan, JC Nelson, and SS Yen, "Effects of replacement dose of dehydroepiandrosterone in men and women of advancing age," *J Clin*

Endocrinol Metab 1994 Jun;78(6):1360–7; G De Pergola, M Zamboni, M Sciaraffia, E Turcato, N Pannacciulli, F Armellini, F Giorgino, S Perrini, O Bosello, and R Giorgino, "Body fat accumulation is possibly responsible for lower dehydroepiandrosterone circulating levels in premenopausal obese women," *Int J Obes Relat Metab Disord* 1996 Dec;20 (12):1105–10.

76. V Bobyleva, et al., "The effects of the ergosteroid 7-oxo-dehydroepiandrosterone on mitochondrial membrane potential: possible relationship to thermogenesis," *Arch Biochem Biophys* 1997 May 1;341(1):122–8.

77. A complete set of references on DHEA is in Julian Whitaker, "DHEA Reference," supplement to *Health & Healing* (June 1992).

78. Low levels of DHEA have been found in women as much as nine years before the development of breast cancer, and many of those with breast cancer have abnormally low levels of DHEA in their blood and urine samples.

79. Michael Murray and Joseph Pizzorno, *Encyclopedia of Natural Medicine* (Prima Publishing, 1991), 53–4, 56, 167, and elsewhere covers the various benefits of digestive aids. This encyclopedia also includes elaborate references, and Chapter 5, "Digestion" (50–56), is well worth consulting on the general issues.

80. M Leuti and M Vignali, "Influence of bromelain on penetration of antibiotics in uterus, salpinx and ovary," *Drugs Under Exp Clin Res* 1978;4:45–48.

81. CD Jennings, K Boleyn, SR Bridges, PJ Wood, and JW Anderson, "A comparison of the lipid-lowering and intestinal morphological effects of cholestyramine, chitosan, and oat gum in rats," *Proc Soc Exp Biol Med* 1988 Oct;189(1):13–20.

82. R Ylitalo, et al., "Cholesterol-lowering properties and safety of chitosan," *Arzneimittelforschung* 2002;52(1):1–7. Chitosan theoretically presents an issue for some individuals allergic to crustaceans inasmuch as these are a common source of the material.

83. K Deuchi, et al., "Continuous and massive intake of chitosan affects mineral and fat-soluble vitamin status in rats fed on a high-fat diet," *Biosci Biotechnol Biochem* 1995 Jul;59(7):1211–6.

84. JJ Marshall and CM Lauda, "Purification and properties of phaseolamine, an inhibitor of alpha amylase, from the kidney bean, *Phaseolus vulgaris*," *J Biol Chem* 1975 Oct 25;250(20):8030–7.

85. P Layer, AR Zinsmeister, and EP DiMagno, "Effects of decreasing intraluminal amylase activity on starch digestion and postprandial gastrointestinal function in humans," *Gastroenterology* 1986 Jul;91(1):41–8.

86. K Kagawa, et al., "Globin digest, acidic protease hydrolysate, inhibits dietary hypertriglyceridemia and Val-Val-Tyr-Pro, one of its constituents, possesses most superior effect," *Life Sci* 1996;58(20):1745–55.

87. EP Brody, "Biological activities of bovine glycomacropeptide," *Br J Nutr* 2000 Nov;84(suppl 1):S39–46.

88. Y Boirie, et al., "Slow and fast dietary proteins differently modulate postprandial protein accretion," *Proc Natl Acad Sci USA* 1997 Dec 23;94(26):14930–5.

89. Michael D Lemonick, "Is the new fat-free fat good for you?" *The Natural Way* 1996 May/Jun:40–45; *Time* (January 8, 1996), 52–61.

90. K Dib, et al., "Effects of sodium saccharine diet on fat cell lypolysis: evidence for increased function of the adenylyl cyclase catalyst," *Int J Obes* 1996;29:15–20; MD Gold, et al., "Aspartame: research update (Parts 1 & 2)," *Smart Drug News* 1995;4(1–2); JE Blundell and SM Green, "Effect of sucrose and sweeteners on appetite and energy intake," *Int J Obes* 1996;20(suppl 2):S12–S17; KM Appleton, et al., "The effects of drinks containing artificial sweeteners or sucrose on food intake following exercise," *Int J Obes* 1996;20(suppl 4):67 (abstract 06-162-WP1).

91. KL Teff, J Devine, and K Engelman, "Sweet taste: effect on cephalic phase insulin release in men," *Physiology & Behavior* 1995;57,6:1089–1095; JR Cotton, JA Weststrate, and JE Blundell, "Replacement of dietary fat with sucrose polyester: effects on energy intake and appetite control in nonobese males," *Am J Clin Nutr* 1996 Jun;63(6):891–6.

92. Simon Y Mills, *Out of the Earth* (Viking Penguin Books, 1991), 273–4; GE Inglett and SI Falkehag, eds., *Dietary Fibers: Chemistry and Nutrition* (Academic Press, 1979), passim; B Ershoff, "Antitoxic effects of plant fiber," *Am J Clin Nutr* 1974;27:1395–1398.

93. Vasant Lad and David Frawley, *The Yoga of Herbs* (Lotus Press, 1986), 138.

94. H Davenport, *Physiology of the Digestive Tract*, 4th ed. (Year Book Medical Publishers, 1977), 255.

95. SB Roberts, MA McCrory, and E Saltzman, "The influence of dietary composition on energy intake and body weight," *J Am Coll Nutr* 2002 Apr;21(2):140S–145S; CL Rock, et al., "Reduction in fat intake is not associated with weight loss in most women after breast cancer diagnosis: evidence from a randomized controlled trial," 2001 Jan 1;91(1):25–34.

96. NC Howarth, E Saltzman, and SB Roberts, "Dietary fiber and weight regulation," *Nutr Rev* 2001 May;59(5):129–39; GS Birketvedt, et al., "Long-term effect of fibre supplement and reduced energy intake on body weight and blood lipids in overweight subjects," *Acta Medica* (Hradec Kralove) 2000;43(4):129–32.

97. Julian M Whitaker, *Reversing Diabetes* (Warner Books, 1987).

98. TM Wolever, "Relationship between dietary fiber content and composition in foods and the glycemic index," *Am J Clin Nutr* 1990;51:72–75.

99. DJ Jenkins, et al., "Effect of a diet high in vegetables, fruit, and nuts on serum lipids," *Metabolism* 1997 May;46(5):530–7; J Cummings, "Dietary fiber and large bowel cancer," *Proceedings of the Nutrition Society* 1981;40:7–14; MAH Alfieri, et al., "Fiber intake of normal weight, moderately obese and severely obese subjects," *Obesity Research* 1995; 3(6):541–546.

100. Jeffrey Bland, *Intestinal Toxicity and Inner Cleansing* (Keats Publishing, 1987), 12.

101. Ann Louise Gittleman with J Maxwell Desgrey, *Beyond Pritikin* (Bantam, 1988), 14ff., 72, passim; Udo Erasmus, *Fats and Oils* (Alive Books, 1986), 287–290. A wonderfully witty and useful newsletter that deals with issues related to essential fatty acids in the diet and with nutrition at large is published by Clara Felix, P.O. Box 7094, Berkeley, CA 94707. On GLA generally, see *The Felix Letter* 58 (1991) and also volumes 57 and 62.

102. TA Mori, et al., "Purified eicosapentaenoic and docosahexaenoic acids have differential effects on serum lipids and lipoproteins, LDL particle size, glucose, and insulin in mildly hyperlipidemic men," *Am J Clin Nutr* 2000 May;71(5):1085–94.

103. KS Vaddadi and DF Horrobin, "Weight loss produced by evening primrose oil administration," *IRCS Medical Science* 1979;7:52.

104. Mary G Enig, *Know Your Fats* (Bethesda Press, 2000); Jane Heimlich, "What the food industry won't tell you about margarine and other man-made fats," *Health & Healing* 1991 October;1(3):6–7. Many of the harmful effects of *trans*-fatty acids have been confirmed clearly and repeatedly in animal experiments. Others have been observed clinically in human populations. It is interesting to note that the Indian Ayurvedic system of medicine traditionally considers highly unsaturated oils, such as safflower oil, to be undesirable as frying oils.

105. TC Fantone, et al., "Suppression by prostaglandin E1 of vascular permeability induced by vasoactive inflammatory mediators," *Journal of Immunology* 1980;12:2591–96; DF Horrobin, "A new concept of lifestyle-related cardiovascular disease: the importance of interactions between cholesterol, essential fatty acids, prostaglandins E1, and thromboxane A2," *Medical Hypotheses* 1980;6:785–800; DF Horrobin, "The regulation of prostaglandin biosynthesis by the manipulation of essential fatty acid metabolism," *Rev Pure Appl Pharmacol Sci* 1983 Oct–Dec;4(4):339–83; DR Tomlinson, "Future prevention and treatment of diabetic neuropathy," *Diabetes Metab* 1998 Nov;24(suppl 3):79–83; DF Horrobin, "Essential fatty acids in the management of impaired nerve function in diabetes," *Diabetes* 1997 Sept;46(suppl 2):S90–3; J Belmin and P Valensi, "Diabetic neuropathy in elderly patients. What can be done?" *Drugs Aging* 1996 Jun;8(6):416–29; KA Bruinsma and DL Taren, "Dieting, essential fatty acid intake, and depression," *Nutr Rev* 2000 Apr;58(4):98–108.

106. JS Fisler and EJ Drenick, "Calcium, magnesium, and phosphate balances during very low calorie diets of soy or collagen protein in obese men: comparison to total fasting," *Am J Clin Nutr* 1984 Jul;40(1):14–25.

107. Those particularly interested in trying the growth hormone release method of weight loss should read Durk Pearson and Sandy Shaw, *The Life Extension Weight Loss Program* (Doubleday, 1986). There are some questionable claims made by Pearson and Shaw, particularly with regard to fructose, but also with regard to GH releasers.

108. One of the best reviews of GH release, and one done by a researcher who is himself published in major scientific journals, is Douglas M Crist, *Growth Hormone Synergism* (DMC Health Sciences, 1991).

109. ER Braverman and CC Pfeiffer, eds., *The Healing Nutrients Within: Facts, Findings, and New Research on Amino Acids* (Keats Publishing, 1986). See also the highly negative reviews of the effects of arginine, ornithine, and the arginine pyroglutamate/lysine combination found in W Nathaniel Phillips, *Natural Supplement Review,* 2nd ed. (Mile High Publishing, 1991).

110. L Cynober, et al., "Action of ornithine alpha-ketaglutarate on protein metabolism in burn patients," *Nutrition* 1987;3:187–91; J Wernerman, et al., "Ornithine alpha-ketoglutarate improves skeletal muscle protein synthesis as assessed by ribosome analysis and nitrogen balance post-operatively," *Annals of Surgery* 1987;206:674–678.

111. W Nathaniel Phillips, *Natural Supplement Review,* 2nd ed. (Mile High Publishing, 1991).

112. J Shabert and N Ehrlich, *The Ultimate Nutrient, Glutamine: The Essential Nonessential Amino Acid* (Avery, 1994).

113. TC Welbourne, "Increased plasma bicarbonate and growth hormone after an oral glutamine load," *Am J Clin Nutr* 1995 May;61(5):1058–61.

114. O Kanuchi, et al., "Germinated barley foodstuff feeding. A novel neutraceutical therapeutic strategy for ulcerative colitis," *Digestion* 2001;63:60–67.

115. DW Wilmore and JK Shabert, "Role of glutamine in immunologic responses," *Nutrition* 1998 Jul/Aug;14(7–8):618–26.

116. Lily M Perry, *Medicinal Plants of East and Southeast Asia: Attributed Properties and Uses* (Cambridge, MA: MIT Press, 1980), 175; YS Lewis and S Neelakantan, "(–)–hydroxycitric acid—the principle acid in the fruits of *Garcinia cambogia* Desr." *Phytochemistry* 1965;4:619–625.

117. W Sergio, "A natural food, the Malabar Tamarind, may be effective in the treatment of obesity," *Med Hypotheses* 1988 Sept;27(1):39–40; AC Sullivan, J Triscari, and JE Spiegel, "Metabolic regulation as a control for lipid disorders. II. Influence of (–)-hydroxycitrate on genetically and experimentally induced hypertriglyceridemia in the rat," *Am J Clin Nutr* 1977 May;30(5):777–84; C Sullivan and J Triscari, "Metabolic regulation as a control for lipid disorders. I. Influence of (–)-hydroxycitrate on experimentally induced obesity in the rodent," *Am J Clin Nutr* 1977 May;30(5):767–76; AC Sullivan, et al., "Effect of (–)-hydroxycitrate upon the accumulation of lipid in the rat. II. Appetite," *Lipids* 1974 Feb;9(2):129–34; AC Sullivan, et al., "Effect of (–)-hydroxycitrate upon the accumulation of lipid in the rat. I. Lipogenesis," *Lipids* 1974 Feb;9(2):121– 8; AC Sullivan, et al., "Inhibition of lipogenesis in rat liver by (–)-hydroxycitrate," *Arch Biochem Biophys* 1972 May;150(1):183–9. The LD 50 given by Sullivan and Triscari for oral administration is 4,000 mg/Kg, which implies that multi-gram dosages are safe for humans.

118. EM Kovacs, et al., "The effects of 2-week ingestion of (–)-hydroxycitrate and (–)-hydroxycitrate combined with medium-chain triglycerides on satiety, fat oxidation, energy expenditure and body weight," *Int J Obes Relat Metab Disord* 2001 Jul;25(7):1087–94; SB Heymsfield, et al., "Garcinia cambogia (hydroxycitric acid) as a potential antiobesity agent: a randomized controlled trial," *JAMA* 1998 Nov 11;280(18):1596–600.

119. SE Ohia, et al., "Effect of hydroxycitric acid on serotonin release from isolated rat brain cortex," *Res Commun Mol Pathol Pharmacol* 2001 Mar/Apr;109(3–4):210–6.

120. D Bagchi, et al., "Management and mechanism of appetite suppression by a novel, natural extract of (–)-hydroxycitric acid," *International Scientific Conference on Complimentary, Alternative & Integrative Medicine Research* (Harvard Medical School), p. 9, Abs. 141, April 12, 2002.

121. M Majeed and V Badmaev, "Bioavailable Composition of Natural and Synthetic HCA." Patent Cooperation Treaty (PCT) International Publication Number WO 02/14477 A2, International Publication Date 23 March 2000.

122. E Racz-Kotilla, et al., "The action of *Taraxacum officinale* extracts on the body weight and diuresis of laboratory animals," *Planta Medica* 1974;26:212–217.

123. "Choline: a conditionally essential nutrient for humans," *Nutr Rev* 1992;50:112–114; JW Daily III and DS Sachan, "Choline supplementation alters carnitine homeostasis in humans and guinea pigs," *J Nutr* 1995;125(7):1938–44.

124. Jeffrey Bland, *Choline, Lecithin, Inositol and Other "Accessory" Nutrients* (Keats Publishing, 1982).

125. VK Babayan, "Medium chain triglycerides and structured lipids," *Lipids* 1987 Jun;22(6):417–20.

126. L Scalfi, A Coltorti, and F Contaldo, "Postprandial thermogenesis in lean and obese

subjects after meals supplemented with medium-chain and long-chain triglycerides," *American Journal of Clinical Nutrition* 1991 May;53(5):1130–3.

127. VC Dias, et al., "Effects of medium-chain triglyceride feeding on energy balance in adult humans," *Metabolism* 1990;39:887–891.

128. *Martindale: The Extra Pharmacopocia*, 15th ed. (W.B. Saunders Company, 1979).

129. GD Foster, et al., "A controlled comparison of three very-low-calorie diets: effects on weight, body composition, and symptoms," *American Journal of Clinical Nutrition* 1992;55:811–817. See also the review of data in Robert Haas, "DHA and PYR: New fat-burning aids for very-low-calorie diets?" *Muscular Development* 1992 Jul:16, 168, 172.

130. GA Vansant, LF Van Gaal, and IH De Leeuw, "Decreased diet-induced thermogenesis in gluteal-femoral obesity," *J Am Coll Nutr* 1989 Dec;8(6):597–601.

131. Michael Colgan, "Yohimbine: New fat fighter," *Muscular Development* 1992 Sept:74.

132. Ibid.; C Kucio, et al., "Does yohimbine act as a slimming drug?" *Israel Journal of Medical Science* 1991;27:550–556.

133. AG Dullo, et al., "Tealine and thermogenesis: Interaction between polyphenols, caffeine and sympathetic activity," *Int J Obes* 1996;20(suppl 4):71 (abstract 08-178-WA1).

134. JJ Ros, MG Pelders, and PA De Smet, "A case of positive doping associated with a botanical food supplement," *Pharm World Sci* 1999;21(1):44–6.

135. T Nikaldo, et al., "The study of Chinese herbal medicinal prescription with enzyme inhibitory activity. VI. The study of mao-to with adenosine 3',5'-cyclic monophosphate phosphosdiasterase," *Yakugaku Zasshi: Journal of the Pharmaceutical Society of Japan* 1990;110(7):504–508.

136. JR Shannon, et al., "Acute effect of ephedrine on 24-h energy balance," *Clin Sci (Colch)* 1999;96, 596, 5:483–91.

137. AG Dulloo, "Ephedrine, xanthines and prostaglandin-inhibitors: actions and interactions in the stimulation of thermogenesis," *Int J Obes* 1993; 17(suppl 1):S35–S40.

138. CM Colker, et al., "Effects of *Citrus aurantium* extract, caffeine and St. John's wort on body fat loss, lipid levels, and mood states in overweight healthy adults," *Current Therapeutic Research* 1999 Mar;60(3):145–153.

139. YT Huang, et al., "Fructus aurantii reduced portal pressure in portal hypertensive rats," *Life Science* 1995;57(22): 2011–20.

140. M Yoshioka, S St-Pierre, M Suzuki, and A Tremblay, "Effects of red pepper added to high-fat and high-carbohydrate meals on energy metabolism and substrate utilization in Japanese women," *Br J Nutr* 1998 Dec;80(6):503–10; TP Eldershaw, et al., "Pungent principles of ginger (*Zingiber officinale*) are thermogenic in the perfused rat hindlimb," *Int J Obes Relat Metab Disord* 1992 Oct;16(10):755–63; T Yoshida, et al., "Effects of capsaicin and isothiocyanate on thermogenesis of interscapular brown adipose tissue in rats," *J Nutr Sci Vitaminol* (Tokyo) 1988 Dec;34(6):587–94.

141. "A Pill that Burns Calories: New Metabolism Boosters," *Longevity* 1992 Nov:12.

142. AJ Gruber, HG Pope Jr, "Ephedrine abuse among 36 female weightlifters," *Am J Addict* 1998; 7, 47, 4:256–61; LP James, et al., "Sympathomimetic drug use in adolescents presenting to a pediatric emergency department with chest pain," *J Toxicol Clin Toxicol* 1998; 36, 436, 4:321–8.

143. CN Boozer, et al., "Herbal ephedra/caffeine for weight loss: a 6-month randomized safety and efficacy trial," *Int J Obes Relat Metab Disord* 2002 May;26(5):593–604.

144. Stephen Langer and James F Scheer, *How to Win at Weight Loss* (Thorsons Publishers, 1987), 16–17.

145. See Elliot D Abravanel, *Dr. Abravanel's Body Type Program for Health, Fitness and Nutrition,* 300–302; also Goodman and Gilman, *The Pharmacological Basis of Therapeutics,* 1397ff.

146. P Paranjpe, P Patki, and B Patwardhan, "Ayurvedic treatment of obesity: a randomised double-blind, placebo-controlled clinical trial," *J Ethnopharmacol* 1990 Apr; 29(1):1–11.

147. K Nazar, et al., "Phosphate supplementation prevents a decrease of triiodothyronine and increases resting metabolic rate during low energy diet," *J Physiol Pharmacol* 1996 Jun;47(2):373–83.

148. M Majeed, V Badmaey and R Rajendran, "Method of preparing a forskohlin composition from forskohlin extract and use of forskohlin for promoting lean body mass and treating mood disorders." United States Patent 5,804,596 issued September 8, 1998.

3: The Anti-Fat Nutrient Weight-Loss Program

1. Julian M Whitaker, *Reversing Diabetes* (Warner Books, 1987), 89.

2. J Ribaya-Mercado, et al., "Vitamin B_6 deficiency elevates serum insulin in elderly subjects," *Ann N Y Acad Sci* 1990;585:531–3; KS Rogers and C Mohan, "Vitamin B_6 metabolism and diabetes," *Biochem Med Metab Biol* 1994 Jun;52(1):10–17.

4: Food Factors

1. MJ Singleton, C Heiser, K Jamesen, and RD Mattes, "Sweetener augmentation of serum triacylglycerol during a fat challenge test in humans," *J Am Coll Nutr* 1999 Apr;18(2): 179–85.

2. TJ Tittelbach, RD Mattes, and RJ Gretebeck, "Post-exercise substrate utilization after a high glucose vs. high fructose meal during negative energy balance in the obese," *Obes Res* 2000 Oct;8(7):496–505.

3. SD Poppitt, et al., "Long-term effects of ad libitum low-fat, high-carbohydrate diets on body weight and serum lipids in overweight subjects with metabolic syndrome," *Am J Clin Nutr* 2002 Jan;75(1):11–20.

5: The End of Dieting

1. The effects of television seem to be dose dependent, that is, the more watched, the worse the effects. CA Raymond, "Biology, culture and dietary changes conspire to increase incidence of obesity," *JAMA* 1986;256:2157–8; WH Dietz, "Gortmaker SL. Do we fatten our children at the television set?" *Pediatrics* 1985;75:807–812.

2. Elliot D Abravanel, M.D., *Dr. Abravanel's Body Type Diet and Lifetime Nutrition Plan* (Bantam Books, 1983) and *Dr. Abravanel's Body Type Program for Health, Fitness and Nutrition* (Bantam Books, 1985); Jeffrey Bland, M.D., *Nutraerobics: The Complete Individualized*

Nutrition and Fitness Program for Life After 30 (Harper & Row, 1983); Deepak Chopra, M.D., *Perfect Health: The Complete Mind/Body Guide* (Harmony Books, 1990).

3. Durk Pearson and Sandy Shaw, *The Life Extension Weight Loss Program* (Doubleday, 1986), 9–10.

4. Elizabeth M Whelan, M.D., and Fredrick J Star, M.D., *The One-Hundred-Percent Natural, Purely Organic, Cholesterol-Free, Megavitamin, Low-Carbohydrate Nutrition Hoax* (Atheneum, 1983), 64–7; Calvin Ezrin, M.D., and Robert E Kowalski, *The Endocrine Control Diet* (Harper & Row, 1990), 8–12.

5. SD Phinney, "Weight cycling and cardiovascular risk in obese men and women," *Am J Clin Nutr* 1992;56:781-782; L Lissner L, et al., "Variability of body weight and health outcomes in the Framingham population," *N Engl J Med* 1991 Jun 27;324(26):1839–44.

6. HB G Hubert, et al., "Lifestyle habits and compression of morbidity," *J Gerontol A Biol Sci Med Sci* 2002 Jun;57(6):M347–5; RJ Garrison and WP Castelli, "Weight and thirty-year mortality of men in the Framingham Study," *Ann Intern Med* 1985 Dec;103(6, pt 2):1006–9; HB Hubert, "The importance of obesity in the development of coronary risk factors and disease: the epidemiologic evidence," *Annu Rev Public Health* 1986;7:493–502.

7. Bruce D Charash, *Heart Myths* (Viking, 1991), pages 1–26; Paul Raeburn, "The great cholesterol debate," *American Health* 1990 Jan/Feb:79–90. Internationally, the whole issue of cholesterol and heart disease is sometimes referred to as "hysteria" within the American medical profession.

8. Calvin Ezrin, M.D., and Robert E Kowalski, *The Endocrine Control Diet* (Harper & Row, 1990), 12.

9. Theodore Berland, "Fast Doesn't Equal Faster," in *The Complete Diet Guide for Runners and Other Athletes,* ed. Hal Higdon (World Publications, 1978), 92.

10. D Halliday, et al., "Resting metabolic rate, weight, surface area, and body composition in obese women on a reducing diet," *Int J Obes* 1979;3:1–6.

11. Ibid.

12. JS Stern, et al., "Weighing the options: criteria for evaluating weight-management programs," The Committee to Develop Criteria for Evaluating the Outcomes of Approaches to Prevent and Treat Obesity, *Obes Res* 1995 Nov;3(6):591–604.

13. George F Cahill, Jr, "Disorders of Carbohydrate Mechanism," in *Cecil Textbook of Medicine,* 15th ed., eds. Beeson, McDermott, Wyngaarden (Saunders, 1979), 2091–2094; Joseph Larner, "Insulin and Oral Hypoglycemic Drugs," in *The Pharmocological Basis of Therapeutics,* 6th ed., eds. AG Goodman, LS Goodman, and A Gilman (Macmillan, 1980), 1497–1523; PA Kern, JM Ong, B Saffari, and J Carty, "The effects of weight loss on the activity and expression of adipose-tissue lipoprotein lipase in very obese humans," *N Engl J Med* 1990 Apr 12;322(15):1053–9.

14. RB Simsolo, JM Ong, PA Kern, "The regulation of adipose tissue and muscle lipoprotein lipase in runners by detraining," *J Clin Invest* 1993 Nov;92(5):2124–30.

15. Norman Brown, "Mood food debate: mind over munchies," *People* section, *San Francisco Chronicle* (September 3, 1992); Richard J Wurtman, "The ultimate head waiter: how the brain controls diet," *Technology Review* 1984 July:42–51.

16. Scott Connelly, M.D., "Nutrients are the key to building muscle and losing fat natu-

rally" in *MET-Rx Owner's Manual*, Scott Connelly, M.D., with Bill Phillips (Myosystems, 1992).

17. PM Suter, et al., "The effects of ethanol on fat storage in healthy subjects," *N Engl J Med* 1992;326:983–87; "Alcohol inhibits fat-burning," *San Francisco Chronicle* (August 24, 1992).

18. PA Kern, JM Ong, B Saffari, and J Carty, "The effects of weight loss on the activity and expression of adipose-tissue lipoprotein lipase in very obese humans," *N Engl J Med* 1990 Apr 12;322(15):1053–9; RB Simsolo, JM Ong, PA Kern, "The regulation of adipose tissue and muscle lipoprotein lipase in runners by detraining," *J Clin Invest* 1993 Nov;92 (5):2124–30.

19. Scott Connelly, M.D., "Nutrients are the key to building muscle and losing fat naturally"; Ann Louise Gittleman with J Maxwell Desgrey, *Beyond Pritikin* (Bantam, 1988), 72; Gary Null, *The Complete Guide to Health and Nutrition* (Delacorte, 1984), 76–78. Durk Pearson and Sandy Shaw in *The Life Extension Weight Loss Program* (Doubleday, 1986; 79ff., 318–320) argue that fructose is both safe and desirable. Yet even they admit that they must take additional copper to prevent unwanted increases in blood lipids, that fructose is more apt to raise urate levels than is glucose in the diet, and so on. (B Buemann, et al., "D-tagatose, a stereoisomer of D-fructose, increases blood uric acid concentration," *Metabolism* 2000 Aug;49(8):969–76.) The studies they cite are usually short-term and do not address the long-term implications of elevated levels of urate (salts of uric acid), pyruvate, and other products of the liver, which imply an increased burden on that organ. For an example of the use of fructose to cause hypertriglycerdemia, see MK Hellerstein, "Carbohydrate-induced hypertriglyceridemia: modifying factors and implications for cardiovascular risk," *Curr Opin Lipidol* 2002 Feb;13(1):33–40; O Ziegler, et al., "Macronutrients, fat mass, fatty acid flux and insulin sensitivity," *Diabetes Metab* 2001 Apr;27(2 pt 2):261–70.

20. JE Swanson, DC Laine, W Thomas and JP Bantle, "Metabolic effects of dietary fructose in healthy subjects," *Am J Clin Nutr* 1992;55:851–856; JC Mamo, et al., "Partial characterization of the fructose-induced defect in very-low-density lipoprotein triglyceride metabolism," *Metabolism* 1991 Sep;40(9):888–93; J Yudkin, "Sucrose, coronary heart disease, diabetes, and obesity: do hormones provide a link?" *American Heart Journal* 1988 Feb;115(2):493–8; J Yudkin, et al., "Dietary sucrose affects plasma HDL cholesterol concentration in young men," *Ann Nutr Metab* 1986;30(4):261–6. For a long list of other complaints linked to sugar consumption, consult Melvyn Werbach, M.D., *Healing Through Nutrition* (HarperCollins Publishers, 1993) 2, 27–28, 33, 47, 96–97, 109, 138–139, 145, 155, 233–235, 266–270, 276–278, 326–327.

21. HR Wyatt, et al., "Long-Term Weight Loss and Breakfast in Subjects in the National Weight Control Registry," *Obesity Research* 2002 Feb 1;10(2):78–82; TA Nicklas, et al., "Eating Patterns, Dietary Quality and Obesity," *J Am Coll Nutr* 2001 Dec 1;20(6):599–608; DG Schlundt, et al., "The role of breakfast in the treatment of obesity: a randomized clinical trial," *Am J Clin Nutr* 1992 55:645–651.

22. KL Teff, SN Young, and JE Blundell, "The effect of protein or carbohydrate breakfasts on subsequent plasma amino acid levels, satiety and nutrient selection in normal males," *Pharmacol Biochem Behav* 1989 Dec;34(4):829–37.

23. KE Powell, et al., "Physical activity and chronic disease," *Am J Clin Nutr* 1989;4 9:999–1006; RS Paffenbarger Jr., et al., "Physical activity, all cause mortality and longevity of college alumni," *N Engl J Med* 1986;314:605–613.

24. Centers for Disease Control, *Morbidity and Mortality Weekly Report* 1992 Jan 24:33–35.

25. *Physician and Sportsmedicine* 1991;19(11):151.

26. James E Klinzing, "Carbohydrates, Proteins, Fat" in *The Complete Diet Guide for Runners and Other Athletes,* ed. Hal Higdon (World Publications, 1978), 44–46, 52 (table of body energy sources); Julian M Whitaker, M.D., *Reversing Diabetes* (Warner Books, 1987), 62–77; JP Despres, et al., "Level of physical fitness and adipocyte lypolysis in humans," *Applied Psychology: Respiratory, Environmental, and Exercise Physiology* 1984;56:1157–1161.

27. DR Dengel, et al., "Improvements in blood pressure, glucose metabolism, and lipoprotein lipids after aerobic exercise plus weight loss in obese, hypertensive middle-aged men," *Metabolism* 1998 Sept;47(9):1075–82 ; JP Miller, et al., "Strength training increases insulin action in healthy 50- to 65-yr-old men," *J Appl Physiol* 1994 Sept;77(3):1122–7; R Pratley, et al., "Strength training increases resting metabolic rate and norepinephrine levels in healthy 50- to 65-yr-old men," *J Appl Physiol* 1994 Jan;76(1):133–7.

28. Interview given to James F Scheer in *How to Win at Weight Loss,* Stephen Langer with James F Scheer (Thorsons Publishers, 1987), 128.

29. JA Anderson and CA Bryant, "Dietary fiber: diabetes and obesity," *American Journal of Gastroenterology* 1986;81:898–906; A Leeds and P Judd, "Dietary Fiber and Weight Management," in *Dietary Fiber: Basic and Clinical Aspects,* eds. G Vahouney and D Kritchevsky (Plenum Press, 1986), 335–342.

30. Julian M Whitaker, *Reversing Diabetes* (Warner Books, 1987), passim; PH Groop, A Aro, S Stenman, L Groop, "Long-term effects of guar gum in subjects with non-insulin-dependent diabetes mellitus," *Am J Clin Nutr* 1993 Oct;58(4):513–8.

31. Julian Whitaker, "New hope on obesity and diabetes," *Health & Healing* 1992 Oct;2(11):4ff.

32. WG Abbott, et al., "Short-term energy balance: relationship with protein, carbohydrate, and fat balances," *Am J Physiol* 1988 Sept;255(3 pt 1):E332–7.

33. MA Ohlson, "Dietary patterns and effect on nutrient intake," *Illinois Medical Journal* 1962 Nov;CXXII(5):461–466.

34. E Cheraskin, M.D., D.M.D., WM Ringsdorf, Jr, D.M.D., and JW Clark, D.D.S., eds., *Diet and Disease* (Keats Publishing, 1968), 28.

35. See the elaborate discussion of the work of Himsworth and others found in Julian M Whitaker, *Reversing Diabetes* (Warner Books, 1987), 27–45.

36. Maria C Linder, ed., *Nutritional Biochemistry and Metabolism* (Elsevier, 1991), 294–297.

37. Calvin Ezrin, M.D., and Robert E Kowalski, *The Endocrine Control Diet* (Harper & Row, 1990), 34–37; *Harvard Health Letter* 1992 Nov:6. A far more elaborate treatment of all these topics can be found in HM Katzen and RJ Mahler, eds., *Diabetes, Obesity and Vascular Disease,* 2 vols. (Halsted, 1978) and TL Cleave, *The Saccharine Disease: Conditions Caused by the Taking of Refined Carbohydrates, Such as Sugar and White Flour* (Keats Publishing, 1978).

38. See Dr. Yeshi Donden, *Health Through Balance,* trans. Jeffrey Hopkins (Snow Lion, 1986), 186. Dr. Donden, a Tibetan doctor, was asked specifically what he thought was the most unhealthful aspect of American life. Part of his answer was this: "I think that although your food in general is very good, you tend to put sugar in everything. It is almost as if you use sugar as most people would use salt; you even put it in hot pepper

sauces. You have gotten used to so much sugar that you just keep eating more and more and more of it. It will induce cold diseases, such as diabetes, as well as rheumatism; it will also make great problems in old age."

39. From *The Food Balance Sheet* (World Health Organization, 1983).

40. DJ Jenkins, "Carbohydrate tolerance and food frequency," *Br J Nutr* 1997 Apr;77(suppl 1):S71–81.

41. Stephen Langer with James F. Scheer, *How to Win at Weight Loss* (Thorsons Publishers, 1987), 8ff.

42. F Nomura, et al., "Liver function in moderate obesity—study in 534 moderately obese subjects among 4,613 male company employees," *Int J Obes* 1986;10:349–54.

43. Langer, *How to Win at Weight Loss,* 35ff.

44. *Experientia* 1983;44(suppl):26–44.

45. Jean Mayer, *Overweight Causes, Cost and Control* (Prentice Hall, 1968), 157.

46. Ann Louise Gittleman with J Maxwell Desgrey, *Beyond Pritikin* (Bantam, 1988), 35–7. Linder, *Nutritional Biochemistry and Metabolism,* 294–297.

47. Berland, "Fast Doesn't Equal Faster," in *The Complete Diet Guide for Runners and Other Athletes,* ed. Hal Higdon (World Publications, 1978), 89–92.

48. See Gittleman, *Beyond Pritikin,* 9–14.

49. Gittleman, *Beyond Pritikin,* 14ff and throughout; Udo Erasmus, *Fats and Oils* (Alive Books, 1986), 287–290.

50. RR Michiel, et al., "Sudden death in a patient on a liquid protein diet," *New England Journal of Medicine* 1978;298:1005–1007.

51. HR Lieberman, JJ Wurtman and MH Teicher, "Aging, nutrient choice, activity, and behavioral responses to nutrients," *Ann NY Acad Sci* 1989;561:196–208; see also note 57.

52. Robert J Blumenschine and John A Cavallo, "Scavenging and Human Evolution," *Scientific American* 1992 October;CCLXVII(4):90–96. The popular name "rabbit fever" is not unambiguous; another form of rabbit fever is actually an infection.

53. See Scott Connelly, M.D., "Nutrients are the key to building muscle and losing fat naturally" in *MET-Rx Owner's Manual,* Scott Connelly, M.D., with Bill Phillips (Myosystems, 1992).

54. Mauro DiPasquale, M.D., "Let the fat be with you: the ultimate high-fat diet," *Muscle Magazine International* 1992 Jul and Sept; "High fat, high protein, low carbohydrate diet: Part I," *Drugs in Sports* 1992 December;1(4):8–9.

55. For those already late in life and suffering from some forms of arthritis or other degenerations characterized by the movement of calcium into the soft tissues, however, this diet may again act therapeutically. See the anecdotal information given by Paul Martin, "Primitive Diets," in *The Complete Diet Guide for Runners and Other Athletes,* ed. Hal Higdon (World Publications, 1978), 170–177.

56. For a general discussion of the role of fats in the body, see Mary G Enig, *Know Your Fats* (Bethesda Press, 2000) and Michael Lesser, *Fat and the Killer Diseases* (Parker House, 1991). Unfortunately, much of the research done in the United States on fats has turned out to be of dubious value due to poor precautions to ensure that the fats used in animal

or even human tests were not already oxidized—rancid—when fed to test subjects. Likewise, most of the laboratory animals used, such as rabbits, do not in nature consume more than 5 percent of their calories as fats, and therefore are arguably genetically unsuited to give results applicable to humans. In rabbits the consumption of cholesterol leads to a lipid storage disease that is not at all comparable to the development of cardiovascular diseases in humans other than those with forms of familial hypercholesteremia—again, a type of lipid-storage disease.

57. A Golay, et al., "Similar weight loss with low or high carbohydrate diets," *Am J Clin Nutr* 1996;63,2:174–8; Richard Weindruch, "Caloric restriction and aging," *Scientific American* 1996;274,1:46–52; N Alméras, et al., "Exercise and energy intake: Effect of substrate oxidation," *Physiology & Behavior* 1995; 57(5):995–1000; SD Poppitt, et al., "Short-term effects of macronutrient preloads on appetite and energy intake in lean and obese women," *Int J Obes* 1996;20(suppl 4):61(abstract 03-138-WP1); BC Bock, et al., "Mineral content of the diet alters sucrose-induced obesity in rats," *Physiology & Behavior* 1995; 57(4):659–668.

6: The Cholesterol Controversy

1. S Ramsay, "Trial of HRT to prevent CHD halted early because of increased harm," *Lancet* 2002 Jul 13;360(9327):146.

2. JA Cauley, et al., "Effects of hormone replacement therapy on clinical fractures and height loss: The Heart and Estrogen/Progestin Replacement Study (HERS)," *Am J Med* 2001 Apr 15;110(6):442–50.

3. M Enserink, "Women's health: the vanishing promises of hormone replacement," *Science* 2002 Jul 19;297(5580):325–6.

4. G Taubes, "The epidemic that wasn't?" Science 2001 Mar 30;291(5513):2540.

5. L Hooper, CD Summerbell, JPT Higgins, et al., "Dietary fat intake and prevention of cardiovascular disease: a systematic review," *BMJ* 2001;322:757–763.

6. L Hooper, et al., "Reduced or modified dietary fat for preventing cardiovascular disease," *Cochrane Database Syst Rev* 2001;(3):CD002137.

7. FB Hu, JE Manson, and WC Willett, "Types of dietary fat and risk of coronary heart disease: a critical review," *J Am Coll Nutr* 2001 Feb;20(1):5–19.

8. WD Rosamond, et al., "Trends in the incidence of myocardial infarction and in mortality due to coronary heart disease, 1987 to 1994," *N Engl J Med* 1998 Sept 24;339(13):861–7.

9. WD Rosamond, "Invited commentary: trends in coronary heart disease mortality—location, location, location," *American Journal of Epidemiology* 2003 May.

10. *The Bantam Medical Dictionary* (1981).

11. SB Hulley, JM Walsh, and TB Newman, "Health policy on blood cholesterol: Time to change directions," *Circulation* 1992 Sept;86(3):1026–9.

12. *San Francisco Chronicle* (November 15, 1991).

13. Harold J Morowitiz, "Hiding in the Hammond Report," in *The Wine of Life* (St. Martin's Press, 1979), 241–245. "It's More Than Just the Wine," in *Alternatives* newsletter, David G Williams, M.D. (1993 June;4[24]:3), citing the recent American Heart Association Conference on Disease Epidemiology and Prevention.

14. JJ Bullen and E Griffiths, eds., *Iron and Infection* (John Wiley & Sons, 1987); ED Weinburg, "Iron and susceptibility to infectious disease," *Science* 1974;184:952, passim.

15. TP Tuomainen, et al., "Increased risk of acute myocardial infarction in carriers of the hemochromatosis gene Cys282Tyr mutation: a prospective cohort study in men in eastern Finland," *Circulation* 1999 Sept 21;100(12):1274–9.

16. Steven Findaly, Doug Podolsky, and Joanne Silberner, "Iron and your heart," *U.S. News & World Report* (September 21, 1992), 61–68.

17. Ibid.; JL Sullivan, "The iron paradigm of ischemic heart disease," *Am Heart J* 1989 May;117(5):1177-88; PA Ward, et al., "Modification of disease by preventing free radical formation: a new concept in pharmacological intervention," *Baillieres Clin Haematol* 1989 Apr;2(2):391–402.

18. M Colgan, S Fielder, and LA Colgan, "Effects of multi-nutrient supplementation on athletic performance," in *Sport, Health and Nutrtition,* ed. F Katch (Human Kinectics, 1986), 59–80.

19. L Pauling and M Rath, "Solution to the puzzle of human cardiovascular disease: its primary cause is ascorbate deficiency leading to the deposition of lipoprotein(a) and fibrinogin/fibrin in the vascular wall," *Journal of Orthomolecular Medicine* 1991; 6(3–4): 125–134. See also Richard M Lin, "Lipoprotein(a) in heart disease," *Scientific American Medicine* 1992 June.

20. Linus Pauling, "Case report: lysine/ascorbate-related amelioration of angina pectoris," *Journal of Orthomolecular Medicine* 1991;6(3–4):144–146. Cf, *N Engl J Med* 1993 May 20; 328(20):1444–56, 1487–89.

21. B Hennig, "Dietary fat and micronutrients: Relationships to atherosclerosis," *Journal of Optimal Nutrition* 1992;1(1):21–23, and other articles in the same issue; M Rath, *Eradicating Heart Disease* (Health Now, 1993).

22. Brian Inglis, *The Diseases of Civilization* (Granada Publishing, 1981).

23. E Cheraskin, M.D., D.M.D., WM Ringsdorf, Jr, D.M.D., and JW Clark, D.D.S., eds., *Diet and Disease* (Keats Publishing, 1968), 315, citing several studies.

24. NM Lamont, "Effect of vitamin C supplementation on black mineworkers," *SA Med Journal* 1976;50:198; and discussed in Rudolph Ballentine, *Diet & Nutrition* (Himalayan International Institute, 1978), 58.

25. Ballentine, *Diet & Nutrition,* 58.

26. Ibid.

27. TL Cleave, *The Saccharine Disease* (Keats Publishing, 1975), 89.

28. GS Berenson, et al., "Atherosclerosis of the aorta and coronary arteries and cardiovascular risk factors in persons aged 6 to 30 years and studied necropsy (The Bogalusa Heart Study)," *American Journal of Cardiology* 1992 Oct 1;70:851–8.

Index

About the Authors

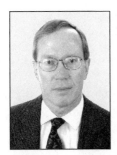

Dallas Clouatre, Ph.D., is a prominent nutrition industry consultant with clients in the United States, Europe, and Asia. He earned his A.B. from Stanford and his Ph.D. from the University of California at Berkeley. A member of the American College of Nutrition and the holder of numerous United States patents, he is a frequent contributor to academic journals and magazines, including *Let's Live, Whole Foods Magazine, Nutrition Business Journal, Vitamin Retailer,* and *TotalHealth,* as well as other consumer- and business-oriented health publications. At *Let's Live,* he provides a monthly column called "How to Buy Guide." He is the author of numerous books, including *FAQ: All About Grapeseed Extract, SAM-e: The Ultimate Methyl Donor, User's Guide to Weight Loss Supplements,* and, with Jesse Stoff, M.D., *The Prostrate Miracle.*

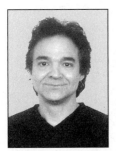

William Karneges, M.Sc., is a health educator and nutritional consultant. He is the author of several nutritional publications, including *Anti-Fat Nutrients* (first edition), *The Memory Test,* and *Never Diet to Lose Weight,* one of the first books to spell out the role of nutrients in altering fat metabolism. He was a pioneer in the development of bottled herbal teas and carbonated fruit juices. He has been interviewed on radio programs throughout the United States, educating millions of people on the transformative power of nutritional supplements. The San Francisco Bay area is his home and work base.